babyfacts

*the truth about your child's health
from newborn through preschool*

ANDREW ADESMAN, M.D.

WILEY

John Wiley & Sons, Inc.

The information contained in this book is not intended to serve as a replacement for professional medical advice. Any use of the information in this book is at the reader's discretion. The author and the publisher specifically disclaim any and all liability arising directly or indirectly from the use or application of any information contained in this book. A health care professional should be consulted regarding your specific situation.

For general information about our other products and services, please contact our Customer Care Department within the United States at (800) 762-2974, outside the United States at (317) 572-3993 or fax (317) 572-4002.

Wiley also publishes its books in a variety of electronic formats. Some content that appears in print may not be available in electronic books. For more information about Wiley products, visit our web site at www.wiley.com.

ISBN 978-0470-17939-0

Printed in the United States of America

10   9   8   7   6   5   4   3   2   1

To my parents—who provided me not only
with guidance and extraordinary opportunity
early on, but also with a lifetime of support
and encouragement . . .

To my wife—for her continued forbearance,
her extraordinary patience, her sage counsel, and
her immeasurable support . . .

and

To my three children—for their consistent understanding
as I worked on this book, for teaching me the things
I did not know as a pediatrician, for making me look
good as a father, and most important, for all of the
joy that they and my wife bring into my life.

Greater riches no man could ask.

The great enemy of truth is very often not the lie—deliberate, contrived, and dishonest—but the myth—persistent, persuasive, and unrealistic.

—President John F. Kennedy

contents

Foreword by William Sears, M.D., xi

Acknowledgments, xiii

introduction 1

The problem: Myth and misinformation, 3

The solution: *BabyFacts,* 5

CHAPTER 1

from milk to cookies 7

the truth about feeding and nourishing your child

- Breast-feeding and bottle-feeding: Facts and fiction
  (and lots of opinions), 8

- Cow's milk: What kind, when, and just how much, 26

- Real food: When milk isn't the only thing on
  the menu, 30

- Sugars: The lowdown on sweet stuff, 41
- Weight gain: What's to blame, and when it's an issue, 46

CHAPTER 2

lights out, kiddo   51

the truth about getting your child to sleep

- Safe sleep: The best position, 52
- Good sleep: From naps to nighttime sleep, from bassinets to beds, 55
- Co-sleeping: When three isn't a crowd, 67
- After the crib: Big-kid beds, night-lights, and things that go bump, 71

CHAPTER 3

from bathtub to booties   77

the truth about keeping your baby clean and comfortable, from head to toe

- Clean and dry: Skin-care tips and bath-time basics, 78
- Baby clothes 101: Dressing your baby, 89
- Safe in the sunshine: Protecting your skin, 92

CHAPTER 4

diapers, disposable training pants, and potties   99

the truth about diapering and toilet training

- Diapers (and a bit of digestion): Don't do anything "rash", 100

- On to the potty: The moment you've been waiting for (and you may have to wait a while), 109

CHAPTER 5

little coughs, big worries 121

the truth about common childhood illnesses and keeping your child healthy

- Colds, coughs, and kids: Treating them the right way, 122
- Fever: Keeping your cool when your child heats up, 133
- Ear infections and sore throats: "Mommy, it hurts when I swallow!", 141
- Conjunctivitis: Don't rub, don't share, and don't panic, 147
- Immunizations: Keeping kids healthy for life, 149
- Allergies and asthma: Know the facts, breathe easier, 154
- Baby teeth: Cutting them, losing them, and keeping them healthy, 164
- Tummy troubles: From colic to stomachaches, 169

CHAPTER 6

growing, growing, gone! 177

the truth about how your child's body and brain develop

- Noggin power: Your child's brain, 178
- Speech and hearing: How your child communicates, 186
- Vision: Bringing the facts into focus, 194

■ Walking: From first steps to first shoes, 200

■ Physical growth: Big, little, and in between, 206

■ Behavior: The good, the bad, and the normal, 210

CHAPTER 7

when accidents happen   223

what to do—and what not to do—when your child gets hurt

■ Head injuries: When (and why) to call a doctor, 224

■ Seizures: What (not) to do, 229

■ Cuts and burns: First-aid care, and when to get
more help, 232

■ Bruises, breaks, and sprains: When sticks and stones
hurt their bones, 234

■ The great (itchy) outdoors: When bugs bite and plants
are pests, 237

■ Stopping trouble in its tracks: Preventing
accidents, 242

Conclusion, 249

Index, 255

Foreword

Love for your baby and your desire to be the best parent you can be make you vulnerable to lots of conflicting advice. Dr. Adesman changes baby myths into baby facts. Parents rely on pediatricians to "show me the science," and that's what you will find in this book. *BabyFacts* exposes troubling myths and misinformation and comforts parents with facts that are backed by science and by Dr. Adesman's own experience as a parent and a pediatrician.

BabyFacts will empower parents to make informed decisions about those daily medical, developmental, and behavioral happenings that are normal in infancy and childhood. In those early years, parenting seems to be a 24/7 marathon of "what to do when . . ."

As a pediatrician and a parent for nearly forty years, I have come up with one piece of time-tested advice for parents faced with on-the-spot decisions, such as what to do when your baby cries at 3 A.M. or when your toddler throws an obnoxious temper tantrum. I tell them: "Get behind the eyes of your baby and ask yourself, 'If I were my child, how would I want my mother/father to react?'" Your reaction will nearly always be right.

Include *BabyFacts* in your parenting library as a resource to help you grow together with your child from infancy through preschool. Enjoy!

William Sears, M.D.,
coauthor of *The Baby Book*

acknowledgments

There are many people who have provided considerable support to me over the years—either directly during my writing of this book or indirectly in giving me the assistance and the opportunity needed to take on this wonderful challenge.

For the past twenty-two years, I have had the opportunity to grow professionally as a developmental pediatrician at Schneider Children's Hospital in New York City. Dr. Philip Lanzkowsky was chairman of the Department of Pediatrics for my first twenty years there. He provided me with considerable support and encouragement to assume projects such as this. His support of my professional development was unflagging. As with many other nonclinical endeavors that I have pursued over the years, I know that this project would not have been possible were it not for Dr. Lanzkowsky's considerable trust, confidence, and support.

In 2006, a new chairman of pediatrics was appointed. Although many people fear change of leadership within a work environment, for me, the more things changed, the more they stayed the same. My new chairman of pediatrics, Dr. Fredrick Bierman, has provided me with the very same level of professional support during his two-year tenure to date. I have been extremely fortunate to have chairmen who consistently recognize the value of projects such as this. Without their support, my dream of writing this book could never have been fulfilled. I am truly indebted to them.

Of course, recognition must go to several others who have provided me with more direct assistance in giving birth to this book. I would like to thank John Silbersack, my literary agent, who had faith in the concept from the very beginning and who gave me the encouragement and guidance that I needed as a new author. I must also recognize the extraordinary efforts of Becky Cabaza, whose assistance with the manuscript was immeasurable. Her stylistic and structural input ensured that the book came to life for the reader. I would like to thank Robyn Feller, who contributed considerably to the medical research.

The final manuscript was reviewed by three outstanding pediatricians. Dr. George Cohen was my first mentor in general pediatrics. His gentle style and warm personality were nurturing and deeply inspiring to me in my formative professional years. Drs. Donna Weiner and Neil Minikes are not only close, long-standing friends, they are exceptional general pediatricians. I am grateful to each of these three physicians for their keen eye and constructive comments regarding the manuscript. I would also like to acknowledge the early support I received from many preeminent physicians—William Sears, Harold Koplewicz, Steven Shelov, Ari Brown, Carden Johnston, Marianne Neifert, Daniel Coury, Harlan Gephart, and Joel Alpert. Each of these physicians recognized the merits of this book when it first was conceptualized. Their enthusiastic praise helped ensure its publication.

Speaking of publication, I would like to thank Tom Miller, executive editor at John Wiley, for recognizing the importance of a book like this, and Christel Winkler, my editor at Wiley, for her assistance in finalizing the manuscript.

As one might expect, writing this book has taken me away at times from other obligations at work and at home. I must thank the professional staff with whom I work within the Division of Developmental and Behavioral Pediatrics at Schneider Children's Hospital—Drs. David Meryash, Ruth Milanaik, Patricia Bigini-Quinn, and Alyson Gutman, as well as our nurse clinician, Patti Hanson. I must give particular recognition to Nancy Alfieri, a special friend, wonderful colleague, and exceptional nurse-practitioner, for all of the day-to-day support that she has given me in my professional life for the past fifteen years. Christine Peck and Angela Trinder also deserve recognition for their administrative assistance in balancing my many work obligations within the Division of Developmental and Behavioral Pediatrics, just as John Brandecker and Steve Friedman have provided me with broad administrative support over the years within our Department of Pediatrics.

Though he no longer is at Schneider Children's Hospital, I would like to recognize Dr. Paul Lipkin; we had the pleasure of working very closely together for many years. He is not only an excellent developmental pediatrician, but also a wonderful colleague. Similar recognition must go to Dr. Harold Koplewicz, who has given me considerable personal and professional support in the many years that I have known him. I truly value the long-standing friendship of both of these physicians.

Finally, I must again recognize the support I receive from my family. My wife, Angela, has provided me not only with the love and support that one would expect in a successful marriage, but with professional guidance as well. As an exceptional pediatric cardiologist, my wife instinctively gets right to the "heart" of the matter. She has not only given support and encouragement for this book from a pediatric perspective, but actually provided me with the initial impetus to write it (since we sometimes would find ourselves with opposing viewpoints on some of the presumed "truths" discussed in this book). As the father of three teenagers, I would not be allowed at the dinner table if I did not acknowledge them as well. They have been consistently understanding of the time I needed to write this book. Moreover, they keep me grounded each and every day—in ways that only teenagers can. For those readers whose children are not yet teens, one day you will understand!

introduction

I'm a parent, like you. I'm also a pediatrician. My young patients are cared for by mothers, fathers, and other loving caregivers who are deeply invested in the physical and emotional well-being of their babies and young children and who—like you, and like me—try hard to make the best decisions when it comes to the health and safety of their sons and daughters.

We are luckier than previous generations of parents because we have such a vast wealth of specific parenting information at our fingertips: books and magazines, Web sites and Internet chat rooms, community groups, experts galore, and the hard-earned wisdom of those parents, grandparents, and friends who were parents before we took the plunge.

But after twenty-four years of practicing pediatrics, and seventeen years of helping my wife raise our three children (though she's also a pediatrician, our kids get the sniffles, too), I've concluded that a lot of information from a lot of different sources often leads to a lot of confusion.

Well-meaning, intelligent parents who are bombarded by conflicting bits of information, with some old wives' tales tossed into the mix, make mistakes, some of them harmful. (And if you ever think it would be great to have a pediatrician in your family, even my family falls prey to myth. My wife—remember, she's also a doctor—lovingly admonished our son to put on his sweater or else he would catch a cold, thereby negating the hard medical fact that colds are caused by a virus; and I recently had to stop myself from telling my adolescent daughter that a popular coffee drink was off limits because "coffee stunts your growth.") Here are some questions, laments, and statements of "fact" I've heard from moms, dads, and other caregivers over the years:

> "Now that summer is here, I've been putting sunscreen on the baby and offering him water to drink. That's okay, right?"
>
> —*mother of a breast-fed four-month-old*

> "We know we shouldn't put our infant to sleep on his stomach, but isn't it okay to let him sleep on his side?"
>
> —*father of a newborn*

"But I've heard vaccines cause autism—I don't want to continue immunizing my child if it means running the risk of a serious disorder."

—mother of a one-year-old

"My daughter touched a hot stove so we put ice on the burn."

—father of a three-year-old

"We play Mozart CDs for our babies. We had read an article about classical music and higher levels of intelligence in infants and children."

—parents of eight-month-old twins

"He isn't toilet trained yet and he's nearly two and a half. Something must be wrong."

—grandmother of a preschooler

The Problem: Myth and Misinformation

Are these parents and this concerned grandparent right? Wrong? Or just downright confused because they have too much—or perhaps not enough—information? Sometimes the mistakes we make in the day-to-day care of our children are harmless. But sometimes these errors can seriously compromise a child's health and safety, or at the very least, cause discomfort, setbacks, and frustrations. Just to take a few of the examples above:

■ *"I've been putting sunscreen on the baby and offering him water . . ."* This mother is partly correct. The American Academy of Pediatrics now considers it acceptable to apply a small amount of sunscreen to an infant under six months of age on areas that cannot be covered by clothing (the long-term effects of sunscreen on infants under age six months are not entirely known), but this is a relatively new development and many parents still believe what those old bottles of sunscreen say on the back—"not for use on infants under six months of age." Toss out the expired sunscreen, for starters, and listen to the latest facts, not outdated beliefs. But as for the water, a breast-fed baby gets *all* the liquid he needs from breast milk. Unless your baby is significantly dehydrated, and your pediatrician directs you to supplement, there is no need to give water, and in fact, offering liquids other than breast milk can interfere with regular feedings and breast milk production.

■ *"But I've heard vaccines cause autism . . ."* Despite the Internet chatter and bad press about vaccines, there is no link between vaccinations and autism. Simply put, immunizations save lives and protect children from disease. In recent years, the mercury-containing vaccine preservative thimerosal (which was removed from almost all childhood vaccines after 2001) was thought to be linked to autism and autism spectrum disorders, but recent studies and research have disproved this theory. There is no vaccine-autism link, and there is no reason to avoid lifesaving childhood vaccinations.

■ *"We put ice on the burn . . ."* Don't reach for ice. If your child sustains a first-degree burn where the outermost layer of skin is only reddened, hold the affected area under cool running water for about five minutes or until the pain lessens. Cooling down the skin is an important first step in relieving the pain and swelling. Ice might seem like a faster way to lower the skin temperature and accomplish these goals, but because even a minor first-degree burn exposes delicate skin tissue, applying ice may actually cause frostbite. Butter is also an inappropriate home remedy. Butter or any other fat or oil-based substance actually traps heat, which can further damage skin tissue.

For years I've been deeply concerned about the misinformation surrounding the care of young children, from the more serious—you would be surprised at how many well-meaning adults still put infants to sleep on their stomachs—to the lighter side of popular myths, which essentially are innocent folklore. As a health care professional, I am not alone in my concern. Many of my medical colleagues are quick to agree that some long-held beliefs can inadvertently harm, injure, or even threaten the life of a young child. At the very least, the prevalence of these myths overcomplicates the joyful, rewarding job of parenting.

The Solution: *BabyFacts*

This book was written to help you separate the parenting myths from the kid realities, from newborns through preschool age, because what you do—or don't do—in the first three to four years after birth can have an impact on your child that lasts, in some cases, a lifetime.

Designed to be easy to use for any busy parent or caregiver, *BabyFacts* is organized into chapters by topic—such as feeding, sleeping, or common childhood illnesses—with each of these chapters further subdivided into more specific areas. Each myth will be followed by the reality and its explanation, which will be full of practical take-aways that you can put to use immediately (or that will set your mind at ease). You'll also see occasional boxes that explore common questions or related myths, or provide more in-depth information on a topic.

I've combed through the latest scientific and pediatric literature, read the recommendations from leading physicians and medical organizations including the American Academy of Pediatrics (which I will refer to as the AAP), sorted through the Internet buzz and the old wives' tales, and have drawn upon my own experiences as a pediatrician and as a parent—who once upon a time was a *brand-new* parent and a recipient of an avalanche of well-meaning (often incorrect) advice, despite my medical degree (and that of my spouse). The result is this book, and I hope it will help you successfully navigate the maze of myth and misinformation.

Note: When I refer to a "newborn," I mean a baby in its first four weeks of life; "infant" refers to the older baby, up to age one; "toddler" refers to the ages of one to three; "preschooler" generally means three- and four-year-olds.

from milk to cookies

the truth about feeding and nourishing your child

My oldest child's first solid food was not an organic apple slice, a calcium-rich cheese stick, or free-range chicken. It was a half-sour pickle. Perhaps after all that milk, she was looking for something with a little zing. One friend had a baby who loved licking slices of lemon and lime. Another had a toddler who preferred "spicy" water (sparkling mineral water or seltzer) over flat, and salad greens dressed with garlicky olive oil. All these children, like millions of others, then proceeded to go through the "picky eater" phase, but managed to survive, thrive, and eventually expand their culinary horizons beyond fish sticks.

Your decision on what and how to feed your child starts before birth, when you are still pregnant and your child is being nourished in the womb. Once your baby comes into the world, you'll choose breast- or bottle-feeding. You'll make decisions on types of milk and formula, baby foods, solid foods, snacks, beverages, and much more. You'll also get lots and lots of advice, funny looks, and criticism if you do things a certain way. But if you can separate out the fiction from the facts, on topics ranging from breast-feeding to food allergies, you'll be able to feed your child with confidence, even if he insists on dropping his spoon from his high chair just to watch you pick it up. Here, then, are some of the most popular misconceptions—and facts to set you straight—about feeding your baby and young child.

Breast-feeding and Bottle-feeding
facts and fiction (and lots of opinions)

myth
Babies who breast-feed very often probably aren't getting enough milk.

reality
The frequency of feedings is not an indicator of whether or not your baby is getting enough breast milk.

the facts
If you are feeding on demand, which many pediatricians and breast-feeding advocates recommend, then you might feel that your baby is constantly at the breast and you may worry

that he's not getting enough milk. But assuming you have developed a steady supply of milk, that you aren't limiting feeding times, and that your baby is latching on to the breast correctly, it's likely that he's simply having a classic growth spurt. The more you feed him, the more milk you will naturally produce for his growing appetite!

myth

If you are breast-feeding, you must always offer both breasts at each feeding for equal amounts of time.

reality

It's more important to let your baby finish with one breast first, even if that means she doesn't take the second breast at the same feeding.

the facts

Each time you breast-feed, you produce different types of milk. *Foremilk* is the initial breast milk that a baby drinks when she nurses at the beginning of a feeding. It resembles skim milk—high in volume but low in fat and calories. As the feeding progresses, the fat content of your breast milk increases and it begins to more closely resemble whole milk. Finally, toward the end of the feeding, your baby drinks *hind milk*, which is highest in calories and fat, and low in volume.

This means that if you switch your baby to the second breast too soon, she may fill up on the lower-calorie foremilk from both breasts rather than obtaining the normal balance of foremilk and hind milk. This may make it harder for her to get the calories she needs to gain weight.

Some mothers offer both breasts at each feeding; others offer one breast per feeding, then switch to the other breast for the next feeding, alternating throughout the day. If you alternate breasts at each feeding, allow your baby enough time to get both foremilk and hind milk.

Can't tell left from right?

You already have a lot to keep track of, and now you have to keep track of whether you offered the left or right breast at the last feeding? You're so tired you can't even remember which is which! Lactation experts recommend a variety of tricks for keeping track, including the rubber band method: If you are offering the left breast, put a rubber band on your left wrist. When you are done with that feeding, switch the rubber band to your right wrist and you'll automatically know which side to feed your baby on first. Eventually, you'll be able to keep track without a reminder like this. The Web sites http://breastfeeding.com and http://kellymom.com contain good information for breast-feeding moms. (*Note:* If you use information from the Internet, make sure it has been vetted by a licensed, reputable health care professional. Always check with your doctor before implementing a major change in your baby's care or your own.)

myth

No spicy foods or alcohol if you are breast-feeding!

reality

You can have a beer with your enchiladas.

the facts

If you're consuming a healthful, balanced diet, you needn't be obsessive about restricting certain foods and beverages from your diet. Even if you make poor food choices, your baby will still extract the nutrition he requires from your breast milk; but chances are you'll feel a lot better if you eat a good diet. So, is it true that if you eat garlic or onions or cabbage, and drink liquor, your baby will have an upset tummy or suffer from the effects of your alcohol consumption?

Some studies have shown that babies get gassy after their mothers eat foods from the cabbage family (like Brussels sprouts, kale, or cauliflower), or that they balk at "garlicky" tasting milk. But unless your infant is truly sensitive and colicky, he can handle a varied diet. It takes about five hours for the foods you eat to pass into your milk supply, so if you're concerned about the "tummy connection," pay attention to what you eat and when you eat it.

As for alcohol, you avoided it during your pregnancy, but now that you're breast-feeding, can you resume drinking an occasional serving of beer, wine, or other liquor? Many doctors agree that no harm will come from occasional or light (not heavy) alcohol consumption—a few drinks over the course of a week, for instance. Very little alcohol makes it into the breast milk supply, especially if you consume food with the alcohol. If you're at all concerned, then breast-feed (or express milk) before having a drink. By the time your baby is ready for his next feeding, you will have metabolized the alcohol (in a 120-pound woman consuming an average drink, this takes about two and a half hours).

There is no evidence that having an occasional alcoholic drink during breast-feeding harms babies permanently; so no need to "pump and dump" your milk if you've had a single drink. However, you may prefer that your baby not be exposed to milk that may contain any alcohol if you suspect he has a reaction to even the smallest amount. In one study, babies who nursed after their mothers ingested a small serving of alcohol sucked more frequently during the first minute of feeding, but then took in less milk in later feedings. Researchers could discern a different odor in the milk of alcohol-consuming mothers, so perhaps the babies drank less because they didn't like the smell of the milk. However, the babies also took shorter but more frequent naps, which suggests that perhaps they consumed less milk because they were sleepy.

What about caffeine? Unless you can clearly connect its consumption to ill effects in your baby (irritability or wakefulness, for instance), you needn't avoid it completely. However, babies are unable to eliminate caffeine from their systems effectively, so it may build up and cause problems for days or even weeks after you've ingested it. Pay attention to your consumption of caffeinated beverages (not just coffee and colas, but energy drinks, certain caffeine-containing cold remedies, and substances like chocolate—though white chocolate has no caffeine) and moderate your consumption accordingly.

What is "nipple confusion"?

So-called nipple confusion can occur when a baby is offered the breast, the bottle, and/or a pacifier within a brief time frame. Breast-feeding and bottle-feeding require two different sets of skills from a baby. With breast-feeding, and with proper latching-on, a baby places her tongue beneath and around the elongated nipple to help create suction and extract milk. When drinking from a bottle, she uses her lips more and places her tongue in front of the nipple to control the flow of liquid. A pacifier uses yet another set of muscles and reflexes. So it's easy to see why a baby who has not yet caught on to breast-feeding could be confused when artificial nipples are introduced too early.

A breast-fed baby can successfully learn to switch back and forth from breast to bottle (this is a practical concern for nursing mothers who go back to work and continue to breast-feed when they are home); she can also use a pacifier to satisfy her need to suck between feedings. There is no science to suggest that pacifiers cause medical or psychological problems. The American Academy of Pediatrics (AAP) recommends no pacifier usage for the first month of life, so that correct breast-feeding technique is established; however, they have also released data that suggests the use of a pacifier in the first year of life, combined with crib-sleeping, cuts the risk of Sudden Infant Death Syndrome. (For more on SIDS, see pages 52–54 in chapter 2.) If you want to discourage nipple confusion, avoid artificial nipples, including pacifiers, for the first few weeks of life until breast-feeding and latching-on is well established.

myth

You must drink milk to make milk.

reality

While getting enough fluid is important, milk consumption is not essential.

the facts

While it would be nice to think that consuming large amounts of milk (especially in the form of a favorite ice cream or shake) automatically ensures a steady supply of breast milk, it's not true. Since you're losing fluids when you breast-feed, it makes sense to supplement them regularly, but water will do the job, too. If you are concerned about your calcium consumption, then by all means drink milk (fat-free or reduced fat are the healthiest choices, and try other forms of dairy or other calcium-rich foods), but there are no set recommendations for nursing mothers on milk consumption. (The recommended daily calcium intake for a nursing mother over eighteen years of age is 1,000 mg, the same as for any other adult.) No mammals have to drink milk to make milk; humans are no exception.

You may have heard that you should drink eight glasses of water a day when you're breast-feeding. There is no research to suggest that that's a magic number (and in fact, the wisdom of drinking at least eight glasses of a water a day has been questioned in recent years by researchers); there is also no evidence that upping fluid intake increases breast milk output. The best advice is to pay attention to your body and drink when you're thirsty.

myth

If you develop an illness or infection or are taking medication, stop nursing.

reality

In most such cases, there is no reason to discontinue breast-feeding.

the facts

If you develop a common infection—whether it's a breast infection (mastitis) or an illness like strep throat or a bad cold—there is no need to stop breast-feeding. In fact, with regard to breast infections, they clear up faster if you continue to feed with the affected breast. Your baby probably already has the same germs that caused you to get sick, and you're actually boosting his immunity naturally by feeding him breast milk. If he does catch your cold, remember that you are providing him with important antibodies that will help him fight the virus. Even if you have symptoms such as fever or coughing, keep breast-feeding and don't worry about passing the infection on to your baby; chances are he already has some form of it, since by the time you develop these symptoms you've been contagious for a day or longer. (*Note:* If you are infected with the AIDS-causing HIV virus, you *can* pass the virus on to your child and therefore should not breast-feed.)

If you take medication, as with any other substance you ingest, a small amount may pass into your milk supply, but in a minute quantity that is unlikely to affect your baby. You can safely take most over-the-counter medications, such as cold and cough remedies, pain relievers (ibuprofen, acetaminophen), and stomach medications, as well as most prescription medications. (With regard to over-the-counter pain relief, since aspirin is linked to the rare but dangerous Reye's syndrome, the AAP recommends that it be used with caution.) In addition to asking your own doctor and pharmacist (remind them that you are nursing), check with your pediatrician if you have concerns about a particular medication that you've been prescribed. Even most antidepressants are usually considered safe for nursing mothers, since most health professionals believe that the benefits of taking the medication outweigh any risks to the child. Breast-feeding experts add that the negative consequences of interrupting regular breast-feeding are greater than the risk of exposing a baby to a minute amount of a drug. (For the latest information on breast-feeding and contraindications, you can go to http://www.cdc.gov/breast feeding/disease/contraindicators.htm.)

myth

If your baby has diarrhea or is vomiting, stop breast-feeding.

reality

You can safely nurse your sick baby.

the facts

If your baby develops a stomach bug and begins throwing up or having bouts of diarrhea, it turns out the best fluid she can ingest is breast milk. If you have an older baby who is already taking solid foods, you may try stopping the solid foods (check with your pediatrician first) to help with the tummy problems, but don't withhold breast milk. With its invaluable nutritional components—its necessary fats, carbohydrates, and proteins as well as its hydrating properties—it's a superior choice over the "rehydrating" drinks you'll find in the baby-care aisle of your local drug store. Even if she can't seem to keep anything in her stomach, she's still benefiting from breast-feeding, and the milk itself, which is extremely digestible, isn't what's making her throw up. Vomiting is a natural reflex that can be triggered when the gastrointestinal tract is irritated. Breast-feeding can help to calm your upset baby and bring her discomfort to an end.

myth

Some babies are allergic to their mother's milk.

reality

No baby is allergic to its mother's milk.

the facts

Some food allergies are very real, but this one is completely false. It is biologically impossible for your baby to be allergic to your breast milk. Some babies may develop allergies to foods their mothers ingest during breast-feeding, including a reaction to the cow's milk proteins found in dairy products. Bloody stools in young infants can be caused by an allergic reaction to cow's milk protein; if this is the case, the condition usually clears up when the nursing mother lowers her consumption of dairy (she may be advised to give up cow's milk altogether). However, it's unusual for a baby to develop allergies or other severe reactions to foods a nursing mother consumes. (See pages 10–12, "No spicy foods or alcohol if you are breast-feeding!")

If someone (other than a doctor) tries to tell you your baby is lactose intolerant, it's most likely not true. Lactose intolerance is highly unusual in early childhood; it is caused by the body's inability to produce enough lactase, the enzyme that breaks down lactose (milk sugar). Most babies have a generous supply of this enzyme from birth and its production does not generally decline until later in life.

myth
Breast-fed infants need water, too.

reality
Breast milk is the only fluid your infant needs.

the facts
Not that long ago, doctors advocated small amounts of water (or formula or sugar water) for a newborn in his first hours of life before breast milk, since there was a concern that the baby would somehow be unable to swallow the colostrum-rich milk. However, we now know that babies are perfectly capable of drinking breast milk as a first fluid, and that because of its easy digestibility and nutritional makeup, it's the best drink you can offer your newborn.

Even in hot weather, or when your baby has a fever, breast milk is still preferable to water. It has all the fluid your baby needs (it is 88 percent water), with vital nutritional benefits that water (or juice or "rehydrating" solutions) cannot offer. Unless your baby develops a medical condition that warrants supplementing with water or other fluids, stick to breast milk as the drink of choice. There is no need to offer water until your baby starts on solid foods (usually at four to six months, the suggested range for most babies by the AAP), when his need for additional fluids will increase. (*Note*: If your infant is bottle-fed, check with your pediatrician on guidelines for offering water.)

myth
You can't get pregnant while you're breast-feeding.

reality
Breast-feeding is not a reliable form of birth control.

the facts
Breast-feeding does provide a temporary, natural type of birth control because the resulting hormonal changes brought on by lactation prevent normal ovulation, provided you are *fully* breast-feeding (absolutely no supplementary liquids or solids plus regular, frequent feedings). If you can't ovulate, you can't get pregnant. However, even though this effect can last for several months, eventually—especially if you are not exclusively breast-feeding, and once feedings become less frequent—your hormonal balance will change and regular ovulation will return. Once your cycle is normalized, you can get pregnant again, even if you are still breast-feeding.

myth

Bottle-fed babies don't bond as well to their mothers as breast-fed infants do.

reality

Babies, no matter how they are fed, and parents have a unique bond.

the facts

If you can't or choose not to breast-feed, you will probably get an earful about how you're missing out on a once-in-a-lifetime opportunity to "bond" with your newborn.

Don't feel guilty. Adoptive parents, parents of infants who were medically unable to breast-feed, and generations of parents who bottle-fed their babies will all tell you that the loving relationships they have with their children are as strong and indestructible as those of their breast-feeding counterparts. There is no reason that you can't turn your bottle-feeding sessions with your baby into warm, relaxing experiences. In fact, if you bottle-feed, other family members and caregivers—both parents, older siblings, grand-parents, friends, sitters—will have the pleasure of getting to know the new baby in a special, one-on-one way.

How you feed your child is your choice. You and your child have a shared lifetime ahead of you, and every day will offer ample opportunities for bonding, long after the bottles and baby clothes are put away forever.

myth

Canned (ready-to-feed) formula is easier for your baby to digest than concentrated formula.

reality

When it comes to ease of digestibility, there is no major difference.

the facts

The real difference between ready-to-feed formula, which comes premixed in cans or bottles, and powdered or liquid concentrate is cost. Ready-to-feed liquid is more expensive simply because it's more convenient. All you have to do is pour it in a clean bottle and it's ready to use, with no need to locate drinking water or to measure and mix. However, many on-the-go parents prefer powdered concentrate because it's more portable. If you're traveling, you can measure single servings into empty, tightly capped bottles and just add water when you're ready. You can make small amounts as you need them and not have to worry about storing (or throwing away) any costly leftovers. And you don't need to worry about a leaky bottle in the diaper bag. Some powdered formulas are even sold in single-serve packets, though it is nearly always cheaper to buy the larger quantity and make up your own single servings. Liquid or powdered, concentrated or not, your baby should be able to digest either form easily. (Some babies reject powdered formula because its texture may differ from ready-to-feed, a problem that can be solved by mixing powdered formula in a blender.)

Formula is either cow's milk–based (the majority of formula sold) or soy-based, or it is a "specialty" formula for a newborn with specific medical needs. Check with your pediatrician to make the best choice for your baby. Be sure to look for a DHA-enriched formula; DHA is a fatty acid necessary for brain growth and development. Nearly all formulas produced in the United States, including store-brand formulas, now contain DHA.

You may also find that your baby prefers one brand over another, concentrate over ready-to-feed, or powdered over liquid. While you may not be brave enough to try a taste test, your little gourmet may have a strong opinion! Some parents try "homemade" formulas to save money or avoid certain ingredients; be aware that homemade or alternative formulas can be very harmful to an infant because they may contain ingredients a baby cannot digest, and they are lacking crucial nutrients a growing infant must have.

myth

The iron in many baby formulas causes constipation.

reality

Constipation is not caused by iron-fortified formula.

the facts

Iron is an extremely important part of your baby's diet, and iron-deficiency anemia can occur if your baby does not get enough of this nutrient. More important, iron is an important nutritional component from a neurodevelopmental standpoint. Mild deficiencies of iron will not cause anemia, but will adversely affect a baby's development. Breast milk contains all the iron a full-term infant needs, but iron supplements are recommended if a baby is exclusively breast-fed (that is, if solid foods are delayed) beyond four months. Premature babies may require iron supplementation early on, since babies in the womb receive their iron stores at the tail end of a pregnancy. The AAP recommends choosing a formula with added iron to prevent iron-deficiency anemia, from birth through one year of age. Iron in commercially prepared formulas is easily absorbed and digested by most infants. Adults often experience constipation when they take iron supplements, which is probably why the erroneous link between iron-fortified formula and infant constipation exists. If your formula-fed baby is constipated, the culprit may be another ingredient in the formula, such as cow's milk protein. The constipation may also be caused by an abrupt switch in types of formula, from formula to cow's milk, or by a change in the number or pattern of feedings. Before you try to resolve the problem by switching formulas or otherwise altering your baby's diet, consult with your pediatrician. Do not remove iron from your growing baby's diet!

myth
Bottles and nipples should be sterilized before every use.

reality
Normal dishwashing is sufficient treatment.

the facts
You may have a vague childhood memory of an adult carefully and laboriously sterilizing baby bottles and nipples, which in fact is what previous generations were instructed to do. However, because of advancements in water purification and the low, safe levels of bacteria in our tap water, it's perfectly acceptable to wash and dry baby bottles and nipples with dishwashing soap and hot water, or to put them in your dishwasher on a normal cycle. If you are in a country where tap water is not chlorinated, if you are using well water, or if your tap water supply has been contaminated or is otherwise unsafe to drink, then you should sterilize bottles and nipples by placing them in boiling water for five to ten minutes. In addition, when you purchase brand-new bottles

and nipples, follow the manufacturer's recommendations for cleaning them before first-time use. Sterilization before initial use may be indicated, but after that you can wash them normally.

myth
Never heat a baby bottle in the microwave.

reality
You can use the microwave, but be cautious.

the facts

You have undoubtedly heard that microwaving your baby's bottle, whether it contains formula or breast milk, is a dangerous practice because the liquid in the center of the bottle can become very hot and can burn your baby's mouth and throat, or because the microwaving process destroys certain vitamins and nutrients and "breaks down" the milk or formula, or perhaps because the bottle itself will explode. Certainly, if you overheat a bottle, or place a nonmicrowavable bottle into the appliance, you can increase the risk of "hot spots" and other problems.

Though many experts, including the AAP, caution against using the microwave, many parents still rely upon it as a common method for heating bottles. If you are going to do this (and I admit, my wife and I did it), take some precautions. And remember, there is nothing wrong with cold or room-temperature milk or formula.

Place an uncapped, microwave-safe bottle of cold liquid—milk or formula, not breast milk (see the box on page 25)—into your microwave on a low-power setting for ten to fifteen seconds to start. (*Note:* This temperature setting and time period may vary for you, but if you're doing this for the first time, start out with the lowest power setting and a very brief microwave time. There are many variables to take into account. You may be using glass instead of plastic, or 4 ounces of milk as opposed to 6 or 8, or your appliance may be highly efficient or not very powerful. Experiment until you get the desired results.) If you are using powdered or concentrated formula, rather than make it up and then heat the bottle, try heating the water only and adding it to the formula.

After you cap the bottle, gently shake it to evenly distribute the heat and then test the temperature of the liquid by shaking a few drops of the bottle onto the back of your hand or your wrist. And of course, the milk or formula should *never* be hot—lukewarm or room-temperature liquid is ideal for most babies; as your baby gets older, you may find that she likes cooler milk (and of course, as time goes by, your child will drink milk straight out of the refrigerator with no preheating). As an added precaution, let the bottle sit for a minute or so and shake it gently once more, before offering it

If you are at a restaurant, instead of asking them to heat the bottle, request a mug of hot water and warm the bottle in it yourself. That way you know it won't get too hot or that it won't be microwaved in an unsafe manner. Similarly, if you are using an unfamiliar microwave, take into account that it may heat up more (or less) quickly than your own, so test the milk temperature carefully before you offer the bottle.

While some parents use specially designed bottle warmers, you can use the warm water method (which is also safer than microwaving)—placing your baby's bottle in a pan or mug of warm water, or running it under warm water from the tap until it reaches the right temperature. If you express and freeze breast milk into special freezer-safe bags designed for that purpose, follow the bag manufacturer's instructions for thawing the milk. Usually this involves thawing the bags in the refrigerator, or under gently running warm water. It's unwise to microwave bottles with disposable plastic liners in the microwave, as you may accidentally weaken the seams of the plastic liners, which could then burst open during a feeding.

Recently a chemical called bisphenol A, or BPA, found in many plastic baby bottles, sports water bottles, reusable plastic food containers, and other food and beverage containers, has come under scrutiny. These plastics, particularly when they are heated, may leach BPA into foods and beverages. When ingested in very high doses, BPA has been known to harm lab animals. Although no conclusive research has been done to determine BPA's impact on humans, there are increased safety concerns. If you have polycarbonate bottles, do not boil, microwave, or place them in the dishwasher. To minimize exposure, avoid clear plastic bottles with recycling code #7 or the letters "PC" imprinted on them. Use glass bottles or BPA-free alternatives instead.

Too hot to handle?

There is evidence that the naturally occurring vitamins and nutrients in breast milk will break down at high temperatures. Rather than risk wasting this precious resource, play it safe and use the microwave for cow's milk and formula only. You may safely use the microwave for heating small amounts of baby food if you follow the same precautions: Start on a very low power setting and mix the food well, testing the temperature before serving. Put the food into a microwave-safe container first, rather than heating the glass baby food jar, which could grow too hot to the touch because of its small size. Do not use polycarbonate bottles or sippy cups in the microwave; choose BPA-free containers.

Cow's Milk
What kind, when, and just how much

myth
Children over one year of age should not be switched to low-fat or skim milk until school age.

reality
You can usually switch to lower-fat cow's milk at age two.

the facts
Do not feed your baby cow's milk before one year of age, since he will have difficulty digesting it, and since it does not contain the crucial nutrients for a baby's first year of life that breast milk or formula offers.

When you start him on cow's milk, choose whole milk. (In some cases, reduced fat 2% milk may be a better choice. The AAP once recommended whole milk up until age two for all babies, but recently concerns about childhood obesity and cholesterol levels compelled them to revise their guidelines. Two percent milk is now recommended for babies who are at risk for being overweight, from age twelve months to two years; at two years, the AAP recommends going from 2% to 1% milk. If you have a family history of obesity, heart disease, or high cholesterol, consult your pediatrician to determine if 2% milk is preferable.) Some reduced-fat or skim milks have higher concentrations of certain vitamins and minerals that could be harmful to children under two years of age. Also, they do not have enough fat and calories for a normally growing baby's needs, and can't provide the necessary amounts of absorbable vitamins A and D. Once your child turns two, however, and with your pediatrician's approval, it's safe to switch to lower-fat or even skim milk.

As our babies grow into children and young adults, we look for safe, easy ways to reduce the amounts of unnecessary fat, cholesterol, and calories in their diets. Switching the older child from whole milk to lower-fat or fat-free milk and other dairy products (and starting an at-risk toddler on 2% rather than whole milk) is a relatively painless step toward teaching them a lifelong healthy habit.

myth

There's no such thing as drinking too much milk.

reality

Too much of any "good" food is a bad thing.

the facts

Milk isn't the perfect food, but for growing bodies, it's a pretty good one. Babies, children, and adolescents (and adults!) all need bone-building calcium. Eight ounces of milk contain 300 milligrams of calcium, which is 35 percent of the recommended daily allowance (RDA) for school-age children. (If your child has been diagnosed with a milk allergy, consult with your pediatrician on other calcium-rich food sources.) With 8 grams of protein, as well as rich supplies of vitamins D and B_{12} (and added vitamin A), and minerals like magnesium and potassium, milk is a healthy choice for most children.

So, how can you possibly take in too much of a healthy food? If your child fills up on unlimited milk during and between meals, he may not feel hungry for fruits and vegetables, meats, and other components of a balanced diet such as whole grains, including iron-fortified cereals. Cow's milk lacks significant amounts of iron, and can even cause iron loss in some children, as it occasionally causes intestinal bleeding. Also, whole milk is high in fat, with 5 grams of saturated fat (8 grams total fat) per 8 ounces. For babies between one and two years of age, this is not a concern; for older toddlers, and preschool and school-age children, this can become an issue if rapid or excessive weight gain is becoming a problem. (See the reality on page 26, "You can usually switch to lower-fat cow's milk at age two," for more information on substituting lower-fat milk for whole milk.)

Milk should be a part of your child's balanced diet, not the focus. The AAP recommends limiting milk consumption to no more than 32 ounces per day for toddlers up to age three. Between ages three and five, 16 ounces of milk provides enough daily calcium for your child.

myth

If you have a daughter, when you switch her to cow's milk, only buy organic to avoid unnecessary hormones that may speed up the onset of puberty.

reality

There is debate over what causes early-onset puberty in girls.

the facts

In recent years, the phenomenon of "early-onset puberty" has made the news, with reports of girls as young as six and seven growing breasts and pubic hair. In an effort to understand why this was happening, researchers looked at dietary causes (among other factors) and concluded that widespread exposure to certain chemicals, food additives, and other substances that were similar in their makeup to the feminizing hormone estrogen could have an impact. They concluded in addition that substances that can disrupt the endocrine system (such as chemicals called "phthalates," found in plastic toys and food containers, as well as cosmetics) could also play a role. (High levels of phthalates were found in the bloodstreams of girls recruited for one study.) Other researchers examined links between high-fat diets and puberty. Ultimately, no single genetic or environmental factor has been pinpointed as an exact cause.

A common growth hormone, rBST, which was introduced in the early 1990s to increase milk production in dairy cows, has also come under scrutiny. Some parent and consumer groups linked the use of rBST as well as other additives in commercially produced milk to early-onset puberty. And many other parents, as well as consumer groups and health professionals, objected to this genetically engineered hormone being added to a food consumed by their babies and children—regardless of gender.

Organic milk is produced without rBST or any other added growth hormones, antibiotics, or nonorganic pesticides. However, it can also be twice as expensive as regularly produced cow's milk, so it may not be an option for many milk-consuming families. If you are concerned about avoiding growth hormone in your child's milk, the good news is that many large commercial dairy producers are now producing regular (nonorganic) milk without rBST (read the label on your milk carton), despite the fact that the Food and Drug Administration has deemed it safe for human consumption.

There is no documented link between early-onset puberty in girls and the consumption of commercially produced, nonorganic milk. You may want to purchase organic milk and dairy products for other reasons, but if you want to avoid rBST, you may be able to find more inexpensive options at your local grocer.

**"But if it's organic, then it's safer for
her to eat, right?"**

Some consumers choose organic foods because they mistakenly believe that if they are organically produced, they are nonallergenic. In fact, some of the most severe allergic reactions in those who suffer from food allergies come from unprocessed foods (made without chemicals, dyes, or additives), such as shellfish, wheat, eggs, and soy. If your child is diagnosed with a food allergy, then you should follow your doctor's guidelines on restricting that particular food, even if it's produced organically.

Real Food
When milk isn't the only thing on the menu

myth
If you have food allergies, your baby will, too.

reality
Your "trigger foods" may not cause a reaction in your child.

the facts
If one or both parents have an allergic tendency, their child will have an increased risk for allergies. But what a child inherits from his parents is overall genetic makeup, not necessarily a specific allergy—be it a food allergy, a respiratory condition like hay fever, or a skin reaction like eczema. (*Note:* Allergy researchers have suggested a link between infant eczema and the onset of asthma later in life. Ask your pediatrician for more information if your baby has been diagnosed with eczema.)

For instance, with regard to foods, if you are allergic to corn, your child may be able to consume corn with absolutely no reaction; however, he may develop an allergy to gluten. In other words, his allergies can manifest themselves in very different ways from your own, or he may never show any symptoms of allergies at all. Don't assume that you or your child's other biological parent is passing along allergies. Food allergies, like other allergies, can develop at any point in your child's life. Generally speaking, genetics can increase a child's risk for allergies, but they can also be triggered or exacerbated by environmental factors, stress, or any other condition that taxes the immune system.

How common are food allergies in children?

We are more aware of allergies in young children than ever before, perhaps because the rate of nut allergies—which can cause severe reactions and death—among school-age children has actually doubled in the last few years, and parents are understandably concerned. A study done by Scott H. Sicherer, M.D., a pediatrician and allergist, documents a percentage increase of peanut allergies in kids in the United States from 4 per 1,000 in 1997 to 8 per 1,000 in 2002 (which translates to about 600,000 kids, experts estimate), though the rate for adults did not see much change. Researchers suggest that the rise (particularly among boys, though no one knows why) may be due to the fact that children are eating peanuts and other nuts or nut butters at an increasingly earlier age, before their immune systems are mature (some pediatricians recommend waiting until age three; ask yours); that more skin ointments and other products are nut- or soy-based; and that roasted nuts, in particular, are triggering the reaction. Many schools have established "nut-free" zones in their lunchrooms, and in some cases, peanut butter is not allowed in school lunch boxes. (Peanuts may be getting a makeover in the future, however, as researchers appear to have developed a new breed of peanut that does not contain the allergens that make eating a PB&J sandwich an impossibility for some kids.)

With regard to food allergies in general, only 6 percent of adults in the United States and only 3 to 4 percent of all children in the United States suffer from food allergies. Many more may have "food intolerance" or "food sensitivities"—adverse reactions like bloating or diarrhea after consuming a particular food—which are often confused with allergy, but which do not involve a response by the body's immune system.

myth

Once a picky eater, always a picky eater.

reality

The young child who rejects variety may grow up to be a famous food critic.

the facts

Just like children, taste buds have "growing pains," too! Don't be discouraged if your toddler or preschooler (or school-age child) prefers plain chicken over herb-roasted, or fish sticks to broiled salmon. She wants the macaroni and cheese, not the homemade pasta with fresh tomato and basil. You may dread trying to find a restaurant when you're on vacation, or at Thanksgiving with the grandparents, because your child is going through a "white foods only" phase. When it comes to getting your child to eat fruits and vegetables, an effort that often deteriorates into a battle, I'm reminded of a child who objected to the color green if it was placed on his plate in any form, and only ate yellow-skinned fruits and vegetables: bananas, corn, summer squash, and of course, the occasional lick of a lemon slice. His pediatrician's response to his mother was the same as mine: At least he's eating fruits and vegetables!

Picky eating is a phase that must be tolerated with patience. Unless your child is failing to gain weight or has a nutritional deficiency, there's no reason to worry, and there's no reason to turn mealtime into a minefield. If you make food into a power struggle or an emotional issue by insisting that your child clean her plate after each meal or by forcing her to eat certain foods, you're doing more harm than good. By making a child finish every morsel, you could be laying the groundwork for overeating. How will she know when she feels full if you keep making her eat beyond that point? And if you stand over her until she tries the garlic-infused side dish, she may grow up despising garlic.

How do you get through this phase, which can last for years? First of all, do a gut check, literally: make sure you and other adults or older siblings in your household are setting a good example by eating a variety of fresh and nutritious foods at mealtime and for snacks. Stay away from empty-calorie junk food (sodas, chips, candy), unless you want your child to develop a taste for it, too. For older kids, offer meal choices whenever you can, but don't turn into a short-order cook. Make meals a pleasure and show that they're a valuable opportunity for socializing. Don't seat your child alone with her food while you disappear into the kitchen or catch up on e-mail, or she'll associate the dinner table with isolation and boredom.

Keep pushing (gently, not forcefully) new foods—don't get stuck in the Chicken Nugget Rut, as you're only reinforcing her self-restricted palate. If you feel that you're getting nowhere in persuading your child to eat a more balanced and varied diet, and you're worried about nutritional deficiencies, speak to your pediatrician about adding a daily multivitamin.

Most of all, don't argue or punish over food, though this is an emotional issue for lots of parents. You are, after all, simply trying to nourish your child. Take comfort in the fact that what a child eats over the course of a single day does not determine whether or not she's eating healthily; instead, a nutritious diet consists of the foods a child consumes over a period of several days. Picky eating is harder on adults than it is on kids! Learning to like new foods is part of growing up and it doesn't happen overnight. When the urge to scold grips you, bite your tongue—and she just may use hers more to taste some new foods and even ask for seconds.

myth

All babies and children should take daily over-the-counter multivitamins.

reality

Prescription vitamins are beneficial and required in some cases, but ordinary over-the-counter supplements are often unnecessary.

the facts

Breast-fed babies get almost all of the vitamins they need from breast milk, as do bottle-fed babies who are fed an appropriate formula (see pages 19–21 for information on choosing the correct formula). In recent years, however, the AAP began recommending supplemental doses of vitamin D. In 2003, the AAP recommended that nursing mothers give their babies

a low supplemental dose (200 International Units) of vitamin D beginning in the first two months of life. However, in
November 2008, the AAP doubled the amount of vitamin D
supplementation recommended based on further review of
available research. The now recommend that all breast-fed and
partially breast-fed infants be supplemented with 400 IU of
vitamin D daily beginning in the first few days of life. Likewise,
infants consuming less than one quart of vitamin D–fortified
formula should also receive 400 IU of vitamin D daily.

Studies show that human milk may not provide enough
vitamin D for newborns and infants, particularly if a breast-
feeding mother lives in a wintry, northern climate where it
may be difficult to get exposure to sunlight (the skin makes
vitamin D when it's exposed to sunlight). The AAP's sugges-
tion for additional vitamin D is also probably in response to
their recommendation that sunscreen—which blocks vitamin D production—be used on all children. (See the box on
pages 36–37 for more information on vitamin D.)

Once your baby is ready to move off breast milk or
formula and on to a diet of cow's milk and table foods, he
may get a less consistently balanced diet. He no longer has
the "vitamin safety net" of breast milk and D supplements,
or D-fortified formulas; if he started solids at four to six
months, an iron-fortified cereal helped to keep his diet balanced. Therefore, your pediatrician may suggest an over-the-
counter children's vitamin, or may prescribe one. However,
vitamins on their own do not provide the body with extra
energy for growth and development. Only the calories present in foods containing carbohydrates, proteins, and fats
provide energy, which is all the more reason to encourage
your child to eat a variety of healthful foods.

Some pediatricians will prescribe fluoride drops for older
babies or chewable tablets for toddlers and preschoolers, which
are often available in combination with a multivitamin. Their
main purpose is to provide a source of fluoride for protection
against tooth decay. Fluoride drops are usually prescribed in

communities where the fluoride content in tap water is low or nonexistent (less than .3 parts per million, or ppm), or if your family drinks bottled water instead of tap water. You can also purchase fluoridated drinking water if this is a concern. (If your baby is older than six months and drinks ready-made formula, fluoride supplementation may be needed since you aren't making the formula yourself with fluoridated water.)

Always check with your pediatrician before offering your child any form of nonprescription supplementary nutrition. Though adults frequently ingest large quantities of popular vitamins or minerals such as vitamin C or zinc, for instance, such megadosing in children is dangerous. If your child is consuming a nutritious, varied diet, he probably won't need supplementation. (*Note:* If your baby was premature or you're breast-feeding and are a strict vegetarian, there are different guidelines for supplementation, which your doctor will advise you on.)

Another dose of (more about) vitamin D

Vitamin D promotes the absorption of calcium, which is crucial for bone development and growth. Without enough vitamin D, the bones don't form properly and are weak, brittle, and malformed (rickets afflicts children who don't get adequate vitamin D).

If you follow the AAP recommendations for additional vitamin D supplementation beginning in the first few days of life (now 400 IU for breast-fed babies and for non-breast-fed infants consuming less than 1 quart of vitamin D–fortified formula per day), you may be wondering at what age you can stop offering supplements and let your child's balanced diet take over and do the rest. Once your child begins taking in at least 1 quart (32 ounces) of D-fortified formula or cow's milk each day, you can stop the extra supplements. The bottom line on the AAP recommendations: Until your baby is getting adequate D from another source, continue with the supplements. Since older children are drinking less milk than in the past, many children may require vitamin D supplements throughout their childhood and adolescence.

In recent years, as the use of sunscreen to reduce the risk of skin cancer has risen, so has concern over the human body's production (or slowed production) of vitamin D. The National Institutes of Health suggests that adults, too, can be at risk for vitamin D deficiency, particularly if they live in cities such as Boston, where there isn't enough sunlight from November through February to aid in sufficient vitamin D production, or in rainy climates like the Pacific Northwest, where cloud cover can block ultraviolet rays. While adults are past the age for rickets if their bones have already developed normally, the bones can soften and weaken in adulthood. Osteoporosis is another concern, because without adequate vitamin D, the body can't absorb calcium. Given the importance of adequate vitamin D status during pregnancy for healthy fetal development, the AAP is now recommending that providers who care for pregnant women consider measuring vitamin D levels in this group of women.

For both children and adults, it's hard to get vitamin D from natural food sources and difficult to balance exposure to sunlight without sunscreen with the risks of skin cancer. Therefore, D-fortified milks and other foods, as well as proper levels of supplements, are often the best answer.

myth
Feed your baby carrots to improve her vision.

reality
Carrot eaters wear glasses, too.

the facts

Carrots are a good food choice, whether you offer them as a snack or as part of a meal. Keep them pureed or steamed to a soft consistency until your child is old enough to chew raw carrots thoroughly. But they're no guarantee that your child will have the eagle-eyed vision of a superhero. True, they are rich in beta-carotene, which the body converts to vitamin A, an important nutrient for good eyesight. In fact, people with night blindness often suffer from vitamin A deficiency, which may be the reason that we associate carrot consumption with better vision.

Unless your child actually suffers from vitamin A deficiency, however, consuming vast amounts of carrots (or other beta-carotene rich foods) will not improve her eyesight. But serve them anyway. They're low in calories and rich in an important nutrient, and they're one vegetable kids usually eat with no fuss.

Perhaps you've been cautioned that a daily serving of carrots will inevitably turn your child's nose a bright orange. While this condition—called hypercarotenemia—is not uncommon among children who eat a lot of orange-colored foods, it's often the palms of the hands that appear to have an orange tint. Hypercarotenemia, caused when the body fails to use up all the carrots' beta-carotene, is harmless and eventually vanishes with dietary modification.

myth

Spinach is a good source of iron.

reality

Spinach is a great source of many nutrients, but iron isn't one of them.

the facts

Popeye had us fooled. The famous sailor man downed can after can of spinach, to be "strong to the finish," and we were led to believe that it was high in iron. The myth goes back to the 1870s, when a Dr. E. von Wolf mistakenly put a decimal point in the wrong place when reporting spinach's iron content; the error was not discovered until the late 1930s, but by that time, Popeye was already taking on Bluto and winning. Spinach, it turns out, has a mere one-tenth of the amount of iron von Wolf calculated.

Spinach *is* an excellent source of vitamins A and E, as well as several important antioxidants, along with half a day's serving of beta-carotene (it doesn't all come from carrots!)— all good for a growing body. (*Note:* Raw spinach has been linked to a handful of dangerous—and fatal, especially for children—outbreaks of E. coli. These outbreaks are rare, however, and are always well publicized by the media and by organizations such as the Centers for Disease Control and Prevention.)

myth

Children should drink fruit juice daily.

reality

There is no Recommended Daily Allowance (RDA) for fruit juice, and too much of a "good" drink has a downside.

the facts

Some varieties of real fruit juice—as opposed to fruit-flavored "drinks" or "punches"—can be healthy choices for your child. Fresh-squeezed orange juice and other citrus juices, for instance, are high in vitamin C, and the commercially available calcium-fortified orange juices provide an extra nutritional boost for growing bodies. Apple juice, with added ascorbic acid as a source of vitamin C, is also an acceptable choice. Mango juice has vitamins A and C, and some vegetable juices such as carrot also have plenty to offer. However, giving too much juice—or the wrong variety—can backfire.

First of all, don't let juice consumption interfere with your child's intake of milk or other more nutritious foods. If he fills up on juice, he won't be inclined to drink milk, which is far richer in nutrition. (See "There's no such thing as drinking too much milk" on pages 27–28 for more on this topic.) The same applies to babies who are transitioning to solid foods, as overconsumption of juice can cause them to feel full and reject iron-enriched cereals and other nutritionally beneficial starter foods. Second, juice is naturally high in sugar and calories. If you get your child into a "juice box habit" at a young age, he may grow up choosing juice over water or lower-calorie alternatives whenever he wants to quench his thirst. Worse yet, if he gets into the habit of wanting a sugary-tasting drink a few times a day, he may indulge in soda more often than you'll want him to. If your child is old enough to eat an apple or an orange, then go for the fruit and cut back on the juice. You'll be giving him more fiber and vitamins and fewer empty calories.

Something as pure and natural as fruit juice shouldn't be complicated, but the AAP does offer some guidelines on juice consumption for babies and children.

- Most infants consume some fruit juice by the time they reach one year of age, but it should be limited to 4 to 6 ounces per day, up until age six years. In addition to potentially interfering with balanced nutrition, too much juice can cause gas or diarrhea.

- Do not offer a baby or young child unpasteurized juice. Because of their still-developing immune systems, they can become extremely ill if they consume naturally occurring bacteria in a beverage such as unpasteurized apple cider.

■ You can dilute white grape or apple juice with water and offer it with food to reduce juice consumption. Many parents who dilute juices from the start find that as their children grow older, they prefer mildly sweetened beverages to very sugary sodas.

Finally, think twice before you lay in a few cases of juice boxes. Though they are convenient for school lunch boxes and for travel, don't let your preschooler or young child have free access. While a medium-sized (6.75 fluid ounces) apple juice box does offer 100 percent of vitamin C, it also packs 18 grams of sugar (the equivalent of more than 4 teaspoons of sugar) and 90 calories. If your child is reaching for another juice box, offer him fresh apple slices and a drink of water instead.

Sugars
The lowdown on sweet stuff

myth
Honey is a better sweetener than sugar.

reality
Though honey is a better choice than refined sugar, never give honey to a baby in her first year of life.

the facts
You may have heard (correctly) that honey can be very harmful to a young baby. In its purest forms (labeled, for instance,

as "100 percent natural, raw, unblended and unfiltered") honey may have some health benefits, ranging from anti-biotic properties to serving as an old-fashioned stomach-calming remedy; however, it can be not only harmful but even deadly to a baby with an immature gastrointestinal system. Honey can contain naturally occurring bacteria in the form of botulism spores, which, when ingested, may cause a toxic reaction in an infant. These spores are usually harmless in most adults, but in babies they are essentially poisonous, causing a reaction within minutes if the bacteria are concentrated enough. In such extreme cases, it can cause paralysis of the muscles involved in breathing, resulting in death.

Even when you purchase high-quality, locally produced, and organic honey, avoid feeding it to your baby for the first year of life; after that, her GI system is more mature and able to handle the naturally occurring bacteria in honey. Botulism is an *extremely* rare illness in infants, but never risk exposing your child to its toxic effects.

Are artificial sweeteners like aspartame safe for my child?

Many parents wonder what, if any, risks there are when offering a child a food or beverage containing an artificial sweetener like aspartame or saccharin. These sugar substitutes aren't just in carbonated diet sodas anymore; they can be found in powdered drink mixes, yogurt, puddings, candy, baked goods, frozen desserts, and many other commercially available products. So, which is better for your child: real sugar, or a low- or no-calorie substitute?

Saccharin, once the market leader, was infamously linked to bladder cancer in rats back in the 1970s. Similarly, a recent Italian study linked aspartame with lymphoma and leukemia in rats. But, the generalizability of these animal studies is often questioned and there is no conclusive evidence that these sweeteners cause similar or other serious health problems in humans. At the same time, these sweeteners have no nutritional benefits, although all mainstream health organizations view them as safe, even for children. For parents of youngsters struggling with obesity, a low-calorie drink flavored with artificial sweetener is often a much better choice than a sugar-laden cola, which packs about 150 calories per 12-ounce can, or a flavored "sports drink" or "energy drink." (Aimed at athletes but often consumed by young children who aren't engaging in calorie-burning sports, these drinks generally have fewer calories than a regular soda, but they are not calorie-free.)

This doesn't mean that your child should have unlimited access to artificially sweetened beverages (or foods) just because they are low in calories, as it may lead to over-indulging and poor snacking habits. Like some weight-watching adults, children may develop an attitude of "It's low-calorie, so I can drink/eat twice, three times, four times as much!" (There are a few recent studies that suggest appetite may even be increased when artificial sweeteners are substituted for sugar!) It might be hard to stop a teenager from drinking multiple cans of diet soda per day (or eating half a box of reduced-calorie cookies); you'll have better odds with a young child. As a parent, you can exert some control over how much and what kind of artificially sweetened beverages and foods your child consumes. You can also make sure your child is offered a variety of healthy drinks, such as water and low-fat milk.

If a child is at risk for obesity, most pediatricians would agree that artificial sweeteners can be useful and practical. ("But it's a chemical," a parent of an overweight child objected when a pediatrician colleague suggested offering diet soda to replace the full-calorie version the child loved. "So is sugar," the pediatrician reminded her.) Finally, consider that a glass of iced, homemade lemonade, flavored with a bit of real sugar and fresh lemon, can be a more satisfying treat than several glasses of the powdered, artificially sweetened version. Sometimes this lesson is lost on the very young, who may be more about quantity than quality. But it's worth trying—those budding taste buds just may prevail.

myth

Sugar causes hyperactivity in children.

reality

It's the birthday party, not the birthday cake, that makes your child "hyper."

the facts

It's hard to dismiss a connection between your four-year-old's consumption of his Halloween candy and his subsequent leaps from the living room couch onto his brother's back. Or your little daughter's wild behavior at a wedding reception, when she runs screaming onto the dance floor after consuming wedding cake and ginger ale. But while ingesting sugar doesn't do your child's teeth or growing body any favors, it's not necessarily what's making him act like a maniac.

Numerous studies have been done on the relationship between the consumption of sugar and hyperactivity, with no significant evidence that the two are related. Despite the science, why does this belief persist? Some researchers believe that it's largely perception. In one study, children and mothers were divided into two groups. Half the mothers were told their children were drinking a sugar-free drink and half were told their children were drinking a beverage with added sugar. The "added sugar" moms rated their children's behavior as hyperactive, while the "sugar-free" mothers viewed their children's behavior as normal. In fact, all kids had been given the exact same drink, sweetened with the sugar substitute aspartame. This suggests that the sugar/hyperactivity belief is a common, ingrained incorrect belief among many parents.

Young children, in particular, are thought to be prone to a condition sometimes referred to as "sugar sensitivity." Although objective studies have failed to confirm sugar sensitivity as a cause for hyperactivity, some parents and professionals believe that if children ingest too much sugar, it can have a negative behavioral effect. Too much sugar is always a bad idea; it can definitely be blamed for tooth decay, is full of empty calories, and in some cases may possibly lead to bad behavior.

Experts suggest we look at the whole situation—not just the food or the drink—that may be causing our kids to go wild. If you only allow your child to have sugar on special occasions, chances are those occasions are celebratory ones where the atmosphere is fun and lively, probably with other children present, possibly at a late hour or otherwise off your child's normal schedule. That environment may well be what's triggering his no-holds-barred behavior. What child doesn't get excited during Halloween or over the holidays, at birthday parties or festive family gatherings? There are many good nutritional reasons to limit sugary treats in your child's diet, but chances are it's not the ice cream sundae that's causing him to grin and run in circles. It's that his much-loved uncle, whom he only sees twice a year, just treated him to a very special dessert.

Weight Gain
What's to blame, and when it's an issue

myth
Sugar makes children obese.

reality
No single food is responsible for a child's unwanted weight gain.

the facts

If you're struggling with a child who is headed for a weight problem, you may be compelled to cut out sugar, but a sweet tooth is not the only culprit contributing to the epidemic of childhood obesity. It is true that sodas, juices, fruit-flavored beverages, and other drinks with a high sugar content are also extremely high in calories. For instance, a child can easily consume several hundred nutritionally empty calories each day if she has a soda habit. Weight gain (as well as tooth decay) is linked to sugary beverage consumption, because it is caused by an excess of calories consumed versus calories expended. If a child is drinking a few servings of regular (nondiet) soda, energy drink, fruit drink, or pure fruit juice each day, adding an additional 300 calories or so, she must burn off those calories or she'll put on weight.

There are many excellent reasons to reduce sugar consumption, but a child can become overweight and be at risk for adult-onset heart disease without consuming sugar-laden foods and drinks if she is taking in nutritionally worthless calories found in junk foods such as chips, or french fries, and most fried foods in general, as well as processed foods like frozen pizzas, fatty and salty luncheon meats, refined bread products, fast food, and many other foods found in grocery stores or school lunchrooms. In addition there are many foods that aren't sweet treats—red meats, high-fat cheeses, foods rich in butter and oil—that aren't nutritionally empty but that can be high in saturated fat and calories and should also be consumed in moderation.

The presence of artificial trans fats—produced through the use of hydrogenated oils found in many common commercially manufactured foods like crackers, baked goods, snack foods, and many fast foods—in our diets is headline-making news, since it raises our levels of "bad" LDL cholesterol and contributes to weight gain. (In some U.S. cities, like New York, local health officials have successfully lobbied to require restaurants to reduce or eliminate trans fats or to clearly post its content for consumers.) The Food and Drug Administration now requires that manufacturers comply with clear labeling of trans fats, and many fast food chains and other restaurants have begun eliminating them. Though we think of heart disease and high cholesterol as adult health concerns, the groundwork for these conditions and for obesity is set in early childhood.

If your pediatrician has determined that your child is overweight (never make this diagnosis without a medical professional), reducing the empty calories in sugary foods is one step toward managing the situation, but look at every aspect of your child's diet. The occasional cookie or glass of chocolate milk may prove to be a better choice than a daily bag of potato chips.

myth
Children outgrow their baby fat.

reality
Baby fat can follow a child into adulthood, but it doesn't have to.

the facts

A fat baby used to be thought of as a healthy baby. This belief had some relevance in centuries past, when malnutrition among children and adults was not uncommon. We also once thought that children automatically outgrew their pudginess, that stout little legs would lengthen and thin out with time and chubby baby faces would develop angular features. But now we know that doesn't always happen, and that children who gain too much weight as babies often have a harder time normalizing their weight—a problem that can dog them into adolescence and adulthood—than babies who fall into a normal range.

As your baby grows into toddlerhood and beyond, he will become more physically active and much stronger, his height will begin to take off, and his "baby fat" may well be history. Annual checkups for your child are especially important, as they offer a way for you and your pediatrician to make sure your child's weight is on track for his height. (Never make a diagnosis about your child's weight and embark on any dietary changes without consulting your pediatrician.)

Pediatricians are increasingly being urged by groups such as the AAP and the Centers for Disease Control and Prevention to review a child's body mass index (or BMI, a body-fat calculation based on height and weight) beginning at two years of age, as BMI may provide a more accurate picture for children who are over- or underweight, or who are at risk for future weight gain. The amount of body fat varies with age (even from month to month) and between boys and girls. Though it is possible to calculate your child's BMI through the same standard calculator that adults use, the results should *always* be interpreted by a pediatrician; for children and teens, age and gender are important factors and pediatricians use a special BMI calculator to take these variables into account.

If there is a weight issue, there are many things you can do to ensure your child achieves and maintains a healthy body weight, starting with offering the right amounts of healthy foods and making sure that he gets enough physical exercise each day, and with making sure that you're setting the right example in your own diet and exercise routines. (Sometimes, the best indicators of a child's future weight are his parents.) Often, simple adjustments such as a daily walk to the playground instead of a ride in the stroller, making a switch to reduced-fat milk, or consuming one less serving of juice, can have a big impact on a little body. Although there's no reason to assume that a plump baby or child will be an overweight adult, if your pediatrician has indicated a concern about your child's weight, ask for specific dietary recommendations and consider a consultation with a licensed nutritionist who has experience working with children.

lights out, kiddo

the truth about getting your child to sleep

There's the old saying that youth is wasted on the young. Given how vigorously some kids fight bedtime (and naptime), one could say the same thing about sleep! Someday, those long stretches spent in bed will give way to barely eight hours of shut-eye and a battle with the snooze buttons on the alarm clock. Until then, though, you can exert some healthy influences on your child's sleep habits . . . and maybe some not-so-healthy influences.

Starting in infancy, my older daughter would not go to sleep unless an adult was in the room with her, and we usually obliged. Soon we realized we'd created not only a beautiful baby girl but also a tiny tyrant. As soon as one of us left the room, she just *knew* it—even when we were perfectly quiet—and we'd have to start the whole get-her-to-sleep routine all over again. My wife and I were doting parents (the pediatrician in us both took a backseat to the parent, we admit), and we paid the price for quite a while.

Contrary to some myths and misconceptions, you can't control precisely how and when your child sleeps, but as you'll learn in this chapter, you can encourage safe and healthy sleep routines—from the crib and into the first "big kid" bed.

Safe Sleep
The best position

myth

It's okay to put your baby to sleep on his side.

reality

To reduce the risk of Sudden Infant Death Syndrome, healthy babies should always be put to sleep on their backs—not on their stomachs and not on their sides.

the facts

Despite numerous studies, the exact causes of Sudden Infant Death Syndrome, or SIDS, remain a mystery. However, there is a very strong correlation between SIDS deaths and the belly-sleeping position, and the medical consensus is that *all* healthy babies, from birth to age one, should be placed on their backs for sleeping. Since 1994, when the government launched a nationwide "Back to Sleep" educational campaign to parents of newborns, the rate of SIDS deaths in the United States has decreased significantly, by more than 50 percent. This is a dramatic and positive development, but SIDS still remains the number-one cause of death among infants between the ages of four weeks and one year.

Babies placed on their sides are less stable; they can roll over from a side position onto their stomachs quite easily (or fall over, when they're too young to roll). Babies were once thought to be safe in the stomach position since it was considered the best way to avoid aspiration of food or milk into the windpipe, and subsequent vomiting and choking. However, all signs, including the SIDS data, point to the back-sleeping position as the safest all-around position. (Though pacifiers can be controversial—see the information on "nipple confusion" on pages 12–13, and on possible dental issues on page 168—their use, combined with back-sleeping, is also thought to cut the risk of SIDS, though the exact reasons are still unknown.)

There are a handful of instances where your pediatrician may suggest that you put your baby to sleep on her stomach or side. For instance, some babies with symptomatic gastro-esophageal reflux, malformations in the upper airways, or other specific medical conditions may benefit from being on their stomachs or sides, though a physician should make the recommendation. If your pediatrician suggests that your baby sleep on her side, make sure you bring her bottom arm forward to prevent her from rolling onto her stomach. (See the last paragraph in the box on page 54 for more on side-sleeping.)

You can safely give your baby daily supervised "tummy time" when she's awake, by placing her on her stomach.

Letting her experience the world from this position can be a fun way to play for both of you, and at the same time it helps her strengthen muscles in her neck, arms, and upper body, which she'll need for pushing up, pulling up, rolling over, and crawling.

Heads up for tummy time!

Tummy time builds muscles and is fun for babies, but it also serves another important purpose. When your baby gets to go on her stomach, the pressure on the back of the skull is relieved. Daily tummy time helps to prevent flattening of the back of the head or asymmetric distortion of the head shape (called "plagycephaly"). These positional skull deformities (admittedly a scary phrase—though generally the conditions go away at around nine or ten months, when babies become more vertical) happen to babies who spend lots of time on their backs.

Some parents think that side-sleeping is one way to avoid flattening. While it's true that these conditions have increased since the "Back to Sleep" initiative began, SIDS is a life-threatening risk and positional skull deformities are not. Here is a much better option than side-sleeping that accomplishes the same goal of avoiding positional skull deformities. Each week, alternate the direction in which you place your baby in her crib. Babies tend to focus toward doorways, so by switching directions you will avoid having your baby lying with her head turned consistently in one direction.

Good Sleep
*from naps to nighttime sleep, from
bassinets to beds*

myth

You can control when and how long your newborn sleeps.

reality

Newborn babies fall asleep when they're ready and wake up
when they're hungry, wet, or upset or because of some other
normal cue.

the facts

Before your baby was born, you probably heard horror stories about the sleep deprivation that awaited you, and the
inevitable advice on how to manage the upside-down world
of newborn sleep patterns. ("Newborn" refers to a baby in
its first four weeks of life.) Someone probably even told you,
"It's never too early to put your baby on a schedule!" And
someone else may even have given you a book or an article
on this topic, all in the name of being helpful.

While you can select a comfy crib, pick out the softest
pajamas, and choose a soothing lullaby, you can't control when your newborn sleeps. He won't fall asleep just
because you put him in his crib. He won't sleep for a
long stretch just because it's eleven at night and you gave
him extra breast milk or formula. You can't "tire out" a
newborn as you might an older child. Your new baby's
sleep/wake pattern is not externally induced; instead, he
follows his own internal cycle. And you can't change it with
your actions. If he wakes up "off-schedule," it's generally
because of hunger, a wet diaper, or sensory stimulation
from noise or motion.

Over the coming months, as your baby grows and as feedings become less frequent and more predictable, you'll gain increasing control over his nap and bedtimes. At night, he'll start to sleep for four to six hours at a stretch, then eventually eight, then ten and longer, and you'll be telling him to get out of bed or he'll miss the bus. But now, while he's a newborn, he's in control. So here's one old chestnut that's not a myth: Sleep when your baby sleeps.

How much sleep does my child need?

Depending on your child's age, her sleep needs will vary, but the short answer to this question is, a lot!

Newborns need fifteen and a half to sixteen and a half hours of sleep a day (though, of course, they won't do it all at once).

Starting at one month, infants sleep slightly less, but still they log about fifteen hours, between nighttime sleep and naps. Over the next few months, they'll continue to settle in to more predictable sleep patterns. (Your role in providing consistency is crucial.)

Between four months and their first birthdays, babies need fourteen to fifteen hours of sleep. Blessedly for you, a good chunk of this is starting to coincide with your own shut-eye time. By the end of the first year, nap time is very predictable. Usually, infants this age nap twice a day, once in the morning and once in the afternoon. Naps can last less than half an hour or up to three hours, depending in part on how long she sleeps at night.

From ages one to three, toddlers need twelve to fourteen hours per day. Naps remain important and beneficial, though their duration and frequency may lessen. By age two, most toddlers won't take a morning nap, just an afternoon snooze.

By age three, they may be done with naps entirely, though some preschoolers, and even kindergarteners—despite "quiet time"—may come home exhausted and ready for a short nap.

Older preschoolers and kids up to age six need between eleven and twelve hours of sleep a day.

myth

Some babies don't need to nap.

reality

All babies need lots of sleep, and naps help them meet their needs.

the facts

If you are frustrated because your baby never seems to nap, you may have someone console you with this comment: "Your baby must be gifted—gifted babies don't need to nap!" This is a common belief among those who support the idea of giftedness from birth, an area where very little conclusive research has been done. It seems to spring from the notion that gifted and talented children tend to be very alert and engaged (as are most well-adjusted "average" children), and grow bored when they aren't stimulated or challenged (as do most kids!). Parents of gifted children may report that when their kids were babies, they always craved stimulation, they grew bored with baby toys and games, and they didn't need to nap. Rare is the baby—especially one with a rapidly developing brain—who doesn't need to nap. A baby may not *want* to nap, or may not nap for as long a period as a parent or caregiver wishes, but those are entirely different issues.

Newborns will sleep when and where they want to (see the reality on pages 55–56, "Newborn babies fall asleep when they're ready. . ."), but starting at about four months, babies up to one year of age settle into regular napping patterns, usually for two naps a day (one in the morning and one in the afternoon), ranging from twenty minutes to three hours. Most toddlers will take one two-hour nap daily. By age three, many children are giving up daily naps, though they'll usually agree to a "quiet time" for a half hour or so, which many day cares and preschools schedule each day.

Naps are important, especially if your baby is not yet sleeping through the night. Make sure you're providing a restful environment for your baby and attempting a consistent napping schedule. The nap patterns above aren't hard-and-fast recommendations, they are guidelines based on the nap habits of most children. However, as in all things, remember that each baby is different. Some will nap for two or more hours once a day, while others may go for less than half an hour several times a day—it's those babies in the latter category that never *seem* to nap, perhaps because their exhausted parents would love to get in a solid block of downtime for themselves!

myth
Newborns sleep soundest in bassinettes.

reality
Newborns have different preferences when it comes to where to bed down.

the facts
Your parents have purchased a gorgeous bassinette for their new grandchild, complete with a gauzy canopy that looks

like something out of a fairy tale. There's only one problem. Every time you put your newborn in it, she screams like something out of the Brothers Grimm.

Some babies simply hate sleeping in bassinettes, no matter how lovely or expensive they are. (Though no studies have been done, these may be the same small souls who detest infant swings; just because you own a particular piece of baby equipment, it doesn't mean your baby will like it, which is why veteran parents say, "Borrow and try before you buy."). These sweet little beds become makeshift changing tables or repositories for stuffed animals or laundry. There are other babies, though, who love sleeping in the close confines of an infant-size bed, and the portability of a bassinette is a real plus since it can be moved from room to room or placed next to a nursing mother for nighttime feedings. ("Co-sleeper" style bassinettes attach to the side of your bed so that you don't even need to get up to nurse your baby; he's within arm's reach, but sleeps safely in his own space.)

You can and should make arrangements in advance for where your new baby will sleep, and newborns generally prefer small, cozy spaces like bassinettes, simple padded baskets, infant seats, or rocking cradles before they graduate to a full-size crib. These spaces are secure and warm, comforting sensations for a baby who's just out of the womb and into the world. However, there are babies who, even in their early weeks, will sleep soundly in a full-size crib, while others will only sleep in their car seats. (I know one desperate mother who quickly discovered her new baby's sleep position of choice for the first few weeks was in his car seat, set inside his crib. I wouldn't necessarily recommend it, but it just goes to show how innovative tired parents can be.) Make plans, but be prepared to be flexible until your baby settles into a full-size crib.

myth

Swaddling is an outdated method for comforting a fussy baby.

reality

Swaddling, when done properly, can be an effective soothing technique.

the facts

Perhaps before you brought your newborn home from the hospital, you observed a nurse fold your new baby up in a blanket with all the skill of an origami artist. Was this just hospital habit or was she doing it for a reason? Veteran practitioners of swaddling (including many a neonatal nurse) swear by its effectiveness in reducing colic and fussiness, as well as encouraging sound sleep, since the confined position created by swaddling reminds an infant of the womb and provides comfort and security.

However, swaddling doesn't just mean rolling your baby up like a burrito (though it's not dissimilar!). If you want swaddling to work, you have to do it properly and safely, so that the arms are wrapped tightly (but comfortably) but the legs are not too restricted or forced into a position that could lead to hip dysplasia. Ask a nurse, an experienced parent or caregiver, or your pediatrician to show you the correct technique, or consult a children's health or parenting Web site with video or photos.

Many studies have found that properly swaddled newborns are calmer and colicky babies cry less; swaddled babies, in general, sleep longer and better. Some parents express concern over the risk of SIDS and swaddling. If a swaddled baby is dressed in warm sleepwear and wrapped in a blanket to the point of overheating and/or is placed in a side- or stomach-sleeping position, the risk of SIDS is increased (a side-sleeping infant could roll over onto his stomach). That is why swaddled babies should be placed on their backs, the position of choice for most babies (see pages 52–54), and should never be wrapped in heavy blankets or comforters. Swaddling blankets should be made of light, breathable cotton fabric (an inexpensive receiving blanket will do)—never wool or fleece. Usually, babies only want to be swaddled for the first few months of life. Do not swaddle a baby who can roll over.

Swaddling has been successfully used for thousands of years, and the humble hand-woven "swaddling cloths" of ancient civilizations have given way to specially designed blankets that come with features like Velcro tabs and special pockets for tucking babies' arms snugly into place. You can go high-tech and buy a blanket that comes with its own instructional DVD or allow your octogenarian grandmother to share her wrapping expertise using nothing more than a rectangle of cotton and your newborn. Either way, you may discover that swaddling is exactly what your baby needs to sleep longer and better—and when he does, you will, too.

myth
A nap in the car seat or stroller doesn't count.

reality
If your child is sleeping soundly, it counts.

the facts
In order for you or your child's caregiver to establish routine nap times, it's best to run errands or otherwise work around your baby's nap schedule so that she can sleep comfortably, soundly, and safely at home, probably in her crib. If you are only meeting the needs of one child, this is usually easy; however, if you have a baby whose afternoon

nap coincides with the same hour that your preschooler needs to be picked up, she may routinely fall asleep in the car on the way to school. Perhaps your older child begs to stay at the playground for a little while, while his baby sister slumbers on. Should you or your caregiver press on toward the calm and quiet of home, or is it okay to let your baby nap in broad daylight, amid the shouts and sounds of a lively playground?

Unless your baby is waking well before her usual nap time is up—for instance, her one-hour nap gets curtailed to twenty minutes because of a particularly noisy environment, like a loud playground, or because other children wake and disturb her—it's perfectly fine to let her nap away from home. As she approaches toddlerhood and becomes less portable, it gets harder to pull off a "movable" nap, and a toddler who has been deprived of a regular nap is usually tougher to manage than an older child who didn't get some playground time.

If you are caring for one child who still naps, and one or more who don't, it can be a juggling act, especially in the afternoons. A nap may be missed entirely or taken while an older sibling has a karate lesson. Naps are important, but sometimes they aren't going to happen under ideal conditions. Don't sweat it, as long as you aim for some regularity most of the time, and *all* your children are getting enough sleep. The second child tends to be the one who usually doesn't wind up with quite as many baby pictures as the first; in most families, she probably won't get as many naps in her crib.

myth

Large babies sleep through the night at an earlier age than small babies.

reality

In this case, size really does not matter. No baby, regardless of size, should be expected to sleep through the night for the first few months of life.

the facts

For most young infants, "sleeping through the night" doesn't translate to the same eight hours that you prize. Instead, it's more like five or six hours, but that's definitely an improvement over the one- to three-hour stints you first endured! The mother of a baby who weighs more than your son or daughter may say that her child is sleeping through the night and that his hearty size is the reason. This idea, which correlates size and sleep, has some roots in a basic fact: older babies who weigh more than younger ones may not wake as often because they aren't demanding as many nighttime feedings as they did in early infancy. However, in a recent study of one hundred babies, ages two to four months and weighing from eight to twenty-two pounds, researchers found no correlation between size and sleep, including which babies were more likely to sleep through the night.

myth

If you keep your baby awake during the day, he'll sleep soundly at night.

reality

If you keep your baby up during the day, you'll have a fussy, tired baby on your hands.

the facts

You may have trouble nodding off at the end of the day if you took a nap, but that's not the case for babies and young children, who still need naps or rest time during the day. Keeping your baby awake is one of many tricks you may hear about for getting him to sleep through the night. (Another popular but erroneous tip is to put rice cereal in the bedtime bottle. For more information, see the next myth.)

Napping and nighttime sleep are two different things and should be kept separate. You can't "tire out" a young baby by not letting him nap; you simply make him miserable, and your day will seem a lot longer! Respect your baby's need for daytime sleep. A nap taken too late in the day can result in trouble falling asleep at night; if that's the case, you may want to adjust the nap schedule, gradually moving naps up by ten or fifteen minutes until you reach your goal. A well-rested baby tends to fall asleep more easily than an overly tired one—just like your adult self when you're "too tired to fall asleep."

myth

Adding rice cereal to a bedtime bottle helps babies sleep through the night.

reality

There's no proof that this method has any impact on a baby's sleep.

the facts

"Just add a little rice cereal to his bottle and he'll be out like a light for eight hours, at least!" Some parents will swear by this technique—adding some rice cereal to the last bottle of the day to guarantee the elusive "sleeping through the night" goal. But, it doesn't work, and in some cases it may be unsafe.

When researchers studied the impact of adding a table-spoon of rice cereal per ounce of milk to the bottles of babies as young as four weeks, they did not notice significantly different sleep patterns from those babies who had cereal-free bottles. Once again, this is a reminder that young babies set their own sleep patterns, and it's difficult, if not impossible, to alter their internal clocks. Parents have fallen for the rice-cereal ruse because they believe that perhaps the additional bulk of the rice cereal will slow digestion, minimize hunger, and therefore prevent a baby from waking up for a feeding. Not only is it ineffective, but if a baby is under four months of age and is given rice cereal, he may be unable to digest its nutrients, and discomfort, if not illness, could result. It's better to stick with a plain old bottle at bedtime and let your baby wake up from hunger, not from a tummy ache.

myth
There is only one way to put your child to sleep.

reality
There are plenty of wrong ways to put a child to sleep, but no single "best" approach that works for all children.

the facts
If this book has a theme, it's that every child is different. That said, every child needs to go to bed and stay there. But what's the best way to achieve that goal? The road to bedtime hell is paved with good intentions. Should you let her cry at night, or go to her side? Rock her to sleep with a bottle? Keep your house as quiet as a church or make a little noise so she doesn't need total silence for sleep? Play soothing music and leave a night-light on? Stay in her room until

she's asleep? And when she's older, can you let her jump into your bed when she's scared? Or should you draw a line in the sand (at your bedroom door) as soon as she can walk?

Whatever method you land upon (and you will find one), be consistent. This is common sense, but common sense has a way of being overwhelmed by the sound of a crying baby. Don't let her cry herself to sleep one night and then rush to her side the next every time she whimpers. Avoid missing bedtimes and naptimes, once she's past the newborn phase and is falling into a more predictable sleep pattern. Resist the temptation to rock her until she goes to sleep in your arms each night; not only is this a difficult habit to break once established, but she will also have trouble falling back to sleep on her own when (not if!) she awakes in the middle of the night. (It's not that you shouldn't cuddle and snuggle with your baby at bedtime—few of us would resist these precious, fleeting moments—but if you set up a routine so that your baby does not ever fall asleep without you, you'll have a long, sleep-deprived haul ahead.)

Establish a good sleep routine when your child is a baby, and stick to a consistent bedtime pattern, making changes to fit her needs as she grows older.

Are you tossing and turning over whether to "Ferberize"?

One of the first questions new parents often have—and one that is a source of controversy and confusion—is whether to "Ferberize" a baby. Named for its creator, Richard Ferber, M.D. (and described in his 1985 classic book, *Solve Your Child's Sleep Problems*), "Ferberizing" became a kind of shorthand for letting a baby "cry it out" rather than going to his side. But as Ferber himself has clarified over the years, that oversimplification of his technique is a misconception (and he never used the phrase "cry it out"). You don't decide one night to just shut the door on your crying child and ignore his distress. Instead, you gradually increase the amount of time that you leave your child alone in his bed, the goal being to get him to fall asleep without your presence. Richard Ferber's "progressive waiting" approach is a detailed and prescriptive plan that unfolds over many nights, even weeks, and that can be modified depending on your parenting style and your child. (For complete details, see the 2006 revised edition of *Solve Your Child's Sleep Problems*.)

Those opposed to Ferber's method, as well as to other "ignoring" strategies, object because it seems callous or unsafe to leave a crying baby or child all alone. But Ferberizing and similar approaches allow parents to have contact with their children and to visually observe them to make sure they are safe. The fact is—and I know from personal experience—that it's really difficult to ignore a crying baby, even for a few minutes, especially if you're a first-time parent. These approaches aren't for every parent, but for some families they work wonders.

Co-sleeping
When three isn't a crowd

myth
You should not opt for the "family bed" (co-sleeping) because it is unsafe.

reality
Co-sleeping, if practiced safely, is an ideal arrangement for some families.

the facts

Parents who practice sleep-sharing, as Dr. William Sears calls it, or the family bed, bed-sharing, or co-sleeping, as it is also known, swear by this nighttime routine, in which a baby or young child sleeps alongside Mom and Dad, starting in infancy. It makes breast-feeding (or nighttime bottle feedings), as well as diaper changes, much easier, and it's a natural way to increase the amount of contact a parent has with a baby. Working parents, in particular, often cite sleep-sharing as a vital part of their bonding process.

This is a largely personal decision that you and your partner should consider before you bring your baby home, and it's not a choice that suits every family. (It is also a cultural preference in some societies—in India, for instance, a large majority of parents and children co-sleep—and Americans with certain ethnic backgrounds may naturally choose co-sleeping because it is a long-held family tradition.)

Although the risk of SIDS is actually extremely low, some earlier studies suggested co-sleeping can be a dangerous practice, particularly with regard to increasing the risk of SIDS. In a well-known study on co-sleeping conducted by the U.S. Consumer Product Safety Commission, which documented 515 accidental deaths over a seven-year period in children under two years old, none of the fatalities was deemed SIDS-related. (Most of the deaths occurred in babies three months old or younger.) Rather, the causes of death included but were not limited to accidental smothering by an adult or by bedding, getting trapped between a mattress and a headboard, or suffocation on a waterbed mattress or other inappropriate surface for an infant. Because of this study, released in 1999, the CPSC recommended that co-sleeping be avoided. However, there is plenty of medical evidence that suggests co-sleeping, when done safely, has benefits including enabling and establishing breast-feeding; lessening sleep disruption for babies and parents (especially nursing moms); and even lowering the risk of SIDS, because co-sleeping babies are more likely to sleep on their backs, not their stomachs.

If you opt for co-sleeping, do it safely, and follow these important guidelines to reduce the risk of accidental suffocation, strangulation, or injury:

- Use a mattress, not a waterbed, couch, or other soft, overly cushioned surface, and remove any cords or ties (such as those on curtains and blinds), which could cause strangulation, from the area. Even fabric ties on nightgowns or other clothing, as well as fabric belts on bathrobes, can pose risks if they are long enough to entrap a baby.

- Put a baby (co-sleeping or not) to sleep on his back, not his stomach or side.

- Avoid heavy or fluffy bedding and pillows and do not place an infant under or on top of such bedding. Use a tight-fitting sheet on a firm surface. Co-sleeping babies should not be overly bundled, as the warmth of a parent's body will contribute to their body heat.

- Do not place a baby between two adults; he should sleep next to one adult (probably a nursing mother, most likely to be sensitive to his physical presence) at the edge of a bed fitted with guardrails (see next bullet). Special co-sleeping bassinets that attach to a regular bed and allow baby and parent to sleep in their own space are another safe option. Do not allow older siblings to sleep with babies; they are less sensitive to the presence of the baby, and the risk of accidental suffocation or injury increases. Limit the number of people in the co-sleeping bed to two parents and one infant.

- Use guardrails constructed with mesh (not slats, in which a baby could get caught and injured) that fits snugly against the edge of the mattress. Pushing a bed against a wall instead of using guardrails is dangerous, as it creates a crevice that could fatally trap a baby. Consider moving the mattress to the floor to reduce injury from falling.

- Babies can get trapped between headboards (or footboards) and a mattress. Consider removing head- and footboards.

- Co-sleep in a queen- or king-size bed. A full-size bed is hazardous because it's too small for two adults and one child—even a small infant—and it's easier for an adult to accidentally roll on top of a sleeping baby or cause injury by flinging out an arm or a leg during sleep.

Do not practice co-sleeping under the following conditions:

- If you are obese: In one study, mothers over 175 pounds had a higher risk of overlaying.

- If you are under the influence of drugs or alcohol or are extremely sleep-deprived: You're far less aware of a baby's presence, increasing the risk of overlay.

- If you are a smoker: There is a link between SIDS and smoking (by either parent), which is not limited to co-sleeping. Do not allow smoking in your house.

Since most deaths in the CPSC study were noted in babies three months or younger, it may be that co-sleeping is safest with babies older than three months.

myth
Co-sleeping with a baby will lead to later childhood sleep issues.

reality
When done properly, co-sleeping should have no negative long-term effect on the quality of a child's sleep.

the facts

Some detractors of sleep-sharing may warn you that once your child is in your bed, you'll have a heck of a time getting her out of it. However, advocates of the family bed report just the opposite. If the transition is handled consistently, children graduate to their own beds and their own rooms with few issues.

You may hear reports of children who repeatedly show up in their parents' bedrooms at all hours of the night, who will fall asleep only in their parents' bed, or who crawl right in without asking, but these kids aren't necessarily co-sleepers having trouble transitioning. These are ordinary toddlers, preschoolers, and young kids with ordinary behaviors, all in search of nighttime comforting and the security that they associate with their parents. In fact, children who are rarely or never allowed in their parents' bed may view it as the ultimate forbidden fruit, which makes them want it all the more. And children who are treated inconsistently—sometimes they're allowed in, other times they're banned, with no real pattern or reasons given—may also have a problem staying in their own beds.

If you practice co-sleeping, make sure you are consistent in your use of the family bed. Don't make it an on-again, off-again practice, but view it as a regular arrangement with all participants on board. For information on helping your child transition to her own bed, see the following myth and reality.

After the Crib
Big-kid beds, night-lights, and things that go bump

myth

When your child is two years old, it's time for a "big kid" bed.

reality

There's no set age for moving a toddler out of a crib and into a regular bed.

the facts

Most parents begin to think about moving their toddler into a bed at around twenty-four months or sometime before the third year, often because another sibling is on the way and the new baby needs a place to sleep. But if an impending birth isn't forcing the issue, there's no hard-and-fast rule on when to transition your child from crib to bed, particularly if he is safe (the mattress is in its lowest position, and he's not climbing over high rails or bringing too many objects into bed with him), comfortable (he still fits nicely and isn't cramped), and sleeping well. Most cribs sold today can be fitted with a low "toddler rail" that can extend its use beyond babyhood. However, one morning you may wake up to find that your child has virtually outgrown his special bed, seemingly overnight!

Your child is old enough to understand that his crib no longer fits and that it's time to move up to the next stage. Here are some suggestions for transitioning into a "big kid" bed.

- This can be a fun and exciting time, particularly if you involve your child closely in choosing a new bed and bedding. Let him go shopping with you and have a vote (although you can draw the line if the NASCAR-inspired bed costs as much as a real car).

- If you are using a hand-me-down, you can still make this an event by letting him pick out new sheets and comforters, or having him help rearrange or redecorate his room. (Make sure that older cribs conform to current safety standards. Visit the Consumer Product Safety Commission Web site at www.cpsc.gov and look for crib safety tips.)

- He may be attached to his old crib and may want to give it a proper send-off, complete with a hug and a kiss. Don't take it away without allowing him to say good-bye to his old friend!

- Don't belittle his crib as something for "babies," or he may feel embarrassed at having slept in it for so long.

- If the crib is going to be used by a soon-to-arrive younger sibling, don't wait until the last minute to start the transition. The process may take a while if your child is resisting, and babies sometimes show up early! Also, your child may feel displaced from his crib by his new baby brother or sister, which could then lead to feelings of anger and resentment. You certainly don't want to jump-start feelings of sibling rivalry over bedding arrangements!

- If your child is particularly attached to the crib, and if you have room, you can set up the new bed and leave the crib until he's ready to give his new perch a try.

- Let your child transfer beloved old security objects— favorite stuffed animals, blankets, or books—into his big boy bed (or her big girl bed) for a sense of ownership.

myth

You must always transition from crib to toddler bed to regular bed.

reality

You don't need to purchase a special transitional bed.

the facts

You already know that the baby furniture industry is a highly lucrative one, at least based on how much money you've already invested in cribs, changing tables, high chairs, and infant seats. Beds are definitely one of the bigger investments you'll make; when you purchased your crib, you no doubt saw a huge array of options, including convertible cribs that grow with your child, converting to toddler beds, daybeds, and even full-size beds. But what if you happen to have a crib that simply has one function: crib? Do you need to buy a low-to-the-ground toddler bed, like the ones you see in all the stores? No. You can easily transition straight to a regular bed, following the guidelines outlined earlier (see the reality on page 72, "There's no set age for moving a toddler out of a crib and into a regular bed."). Save your money for your child's next big transitional object—when she goes from tricycle to two-wheeler.

myth
Don't put your child to bed with a light on.

reality
There's no harm done if your child needs light to sleep.

the facts
The use of a night-light or dim lamp, even an overhead light on a dimmer switch, is often a great source of comfort to preschoolers and young children who are going through an "afraid of the dark" phase. It's not uncommon for once-hearty sleepers to suddenly develop a fear of monsters under the bed (see the box on pages 75–76), in the closet, or in the corner, often at around age two or three. This can last for a few years (or it may not happen at all), and a little bit of light can go a long way to calm a child's fears. It was once thought that the use of a night-light caused nearsightedness, since the eyes would then strain to see in the dimness, but

this idea has been discounted by the medical profession. In fact, babies and young children may actually improve their abilities to focus with a night-light in the room. Young babies can strengthen hand-eye coordination when they are lying in dim lights beneath a mobile or other toys they may try to reach. (Crib mobiles should be hung well out of a baby's reach and should be removed from his bed once he can push himself up on his hands and knees). Light may bother *you* when you're trying to sleep, but it may be very the thing that helps your child get some shut-eye.

The monster under the bed: Nightmares and night terrors

Starting at around age two, toddlers may start to have bad dreams brought on by something they saw during the course of their busy day. Perhaps they saw something on television that stuck with them, or saw an illustration in a picture book that took on a life of its own. It's very difficult to explain to a scared and sleepy two-year-old that the green cat with the long teeth that was chasing him was "just a dream." At this tender age, children are way too young to grasp the concept of an imagination, so everything seems like reality. Don't tell your child, "There's nothing to be afraid of," and expect him to accept that and go right back to sleep. (Think back—did that line ever work for you when your parents tried it?) The best thing is to let your child tell you what scared him, comfort him with a hug or two, and help him relax and get resettled for sleep.

Between the ages of two and four, bad dreams are not uncommon, particularly as children have more exposure to new books and videos, toys, or games, more experiences at preschool or day care, and other new influences. Their world is expanding, and so is the stuff of dreams (and nightmares). The neighbor dressed in black whom your child saw that morning becomes a witch twelve hours later. The daytime game of hide-and-seek becomes scary in a dream, when Mommy or Daddy is nowhere to be found. Again, don't dismiss your child's fears out of hand. You can't stop your child from having bad dreams, but if he is upset by one, take some time to listen and to comfort him.

Some preschoolers will suffer from "night terrors," which are different from nightmares and more unusual. Children will appear to be awake (their eyes are open) and will act terrified of something only they can see. They will cry, kick, and scream, but despite all this activity, they are caught somewhere between sleep and being fully awake. They will have no memory of the episode in the morning. Children usually outgrow the night-terror stage, but if the incidents occur frequently enough to interrupt your child's sleep on a regular basis, talk to your pediatrician. Behaviors like night terrors, insomnia (yes, children can have insomnia), and sleepwalking do not mean that a child is emotionally disturbed.

Was your baby born with a sprinkling of tiny white bumps across the nose, cheeks, or chin? Half of all babies are born with this condition, called "milia," which is a result of ordinary skin gland secretions. It will go away in a few weeks. Another common newborn skin condition is called "erythema toxicum," also known as ETN, a blotchy red rash that often erupts within a day or two after birth. Like milia, ETN affects about half of all babies; this harmless rash disappears without treatment in about one week.

Baby acne, which shows up after the milia goes away (at about four to five weeks), is more noticeable, with red pimples that occur on the cheeks and forehead. During pregnancy, a mother's hormones pass across the placenta to the baby; this is a beneficial process, as it stimulates growth (in a baby's lungs, for instance). However, it also stimulates oil production, which can set off breakouts of acne till up to six months of age. It is not cause for concern, as it's a normal skin condition, but it can be made worse if the affected skin comes into contact with spit-up milk or saliva, or in some cases with bedding that has been washed with harsh detergents. You can alleviate it somewhat by gently washing the face each day with a mild baby soap. However, if it persists beyond six months, ask your pediatrician if it should be treated.

Some babies get rashes such as miliaria (though this word sounds similar to "milia," these small clear or red bumps filled with fluid are a different condition), or pustular melanosis (which starts as blisters that dry out and leave dark, freckle-like spots). Both of these conditions disappear.

In warm, especially humid weather (even in winter if they are overdressed) babies can get heat rash, which is actually a variety of miliaria (miliaria rubra—named for the red bumps it produces, as opposed to miliaria crystallina, for the clear bumps). Perspiration is trapped beneath the skin and collects in the tiny bumps, which then burst to release the perspiration (the prickly sensation this rash causes is why it's also known as "prickly heat"). Usually heat rash, which can be itchy, goes away shortly after the skin is cooled down, but it can last for two or three days. If the weather is hot, make sure your baby isn't overdressed (choose light, loose-fitting clothing), and don't put any oils, lotions, or ointments on the bumps, as you'll trap the heat and worsen the condition. Keeping your baby cool and dry usually is enough to send the heat rash on its way. Call your pediatrician if the rash persists or if your baby has a fever. Heat rash combined with fever could indicate other conditions.

If your baby has any rash that does not clear up on its own or seems to be causing discomfort, point it out to your pediatrician.

myth

Birthmarks appear at birth and are permanent.

reality

Birthmarks come in many varieties and can be present at birth, can show up later, can vanish, or can be permanent.

the facts

Not all so-called birthmarks are present at birth, and most are not serious.

"Salmon patches" are perhaps the most common of birthmarks—dark pink patches on the bridge of the nose and forehead ("angel's kiss"), the eyelids, or the back of the head and neck ("stork bite"). These marks are dilated capillaries that are leftovers of fetal blood circulation; the still-red skin shows how the blood vessels developed in a fetus. All babies have them in the womb, and some marks fade shortly after birth while others may remain for life (particularly those at the nape of the neck).

Myths abound about why babies are born with birthmarks, such as this one: A baby with a brown "café au lait" mark had a mom who drank too much coffee or had unfulfilled cravings. None of these myths is true, since birthmarks are simply a part of fetal development. Some may show up after birth, such as "strawberry" hemangiomas, composed of raised, dilated blood vessels. A strawberry hemangioma may be barely visible at birth, its only evidence a rough red spot. Then, as a baby grows, the hemangioma grows, but gradually it will shrink and disappear, usually by age five or six, typically without any treatment. (Hemangiomas that occur around the eyes or mouth area should be monitored.) Birthmarks that don't fade, such as port wine stains, can be treated later in life.

If you notice a new birthmark on your child, point it out to your pediatrician for confirmation that it's a harmless spot—that is usually the case. Always ask about any birthmarks that appear to change in shape, color, or texture.

myth
Newborns should be bathed daily.

reality
Babies don't need daily baths, nor is it good for their skin.

the facts
If you're a first-time parent, you may be understandably nervous about bathing your delicate newborn, and you may want to put off a tub bath (as opposed to a sponge bath) for as long as possible; but your mother is urging you to give

her grandchild a regular bath, as she bathed her own babies daily (and used plenty of baby powder afterward—see the box on pages 88–89 on powder use). Grandma loves to cuddle a sweet-smelling bundle, but unless your baby is truly dirty (or smells like spilt milk—or worse!), you don't need to bathe him more than two or three times a week during his first year. Once he's a busy toddler and getting into finger paints, spaghetti dinners, and mud pies, then you can bathe him more often (particularly if he comes to love bath time, as many babies do). Bathing removes moisture from the skin, so if you're overbathing your child, his skin can become dry and irritated.

You can use a mild soap and shampoo even on a newborn, but you may want to test it on a small patch of your baby's skin to make sure he's not sensitive. (You can also opt for plain warm water for a newborn, and no soap or shampoo unless the skin or scalp is dirty.) If your baby has cradle cap (see the box "Should you treat cradle cap?" on page 85), a mild shampoo and very gentle brushing with a soft washcloth will help remove the scaling. There is some evidence that sitting in bathwater containing shampoo can cause urinary tract irritation, so shampooing is often best done at the end of the tub bath.

As long as you keep your baby's diaper area clean, as well as the neck area where milk or spit-up may collect, and any other skin folds or creases where perspiration and oils may naturally accumulate, your baby will stay fairly clean between baths, whether you do them every other day or go for longer spells (which you may want to do in the winter months). Sponge baths dry out the skin less than tub baths, so if dryness is a concern, you can try a combination of sponge- and tub-bathing.

Most pediatricians will recommend that you wait until the umbilical stump has fallen off (see the box on page 83) and the wound has healed, and that a circumcision has healed, before you immerse your baby in a tub bath, to reduce the risk of infection. But in most cases, if healing is progressing normally and if your pediatrician agrees, you can do a tub bath. However, this means you'll be tub-bathing a newborn in his first days or weeks at home; this probably isn't necessary just yet if you're doing sponge baths. And if you're a first-time parent and you're nervous about tub bathing, why add this level of stress?

Stumped by the umbilical cord? Let nature take its course, with a little help from you.

The umbilical cord stump, which can look gruesome to first-time parents, really will fall off after it dries out. The two watchwords are *clean* and *dry*. If the area is dirty or sticky, you can use soap and water to gently clean the stump. Dry carefully. Keep the stump exposed to the air (fold the diaper down so that the cord is not covered) to help the process along. Never pull on the cord, no matter how gently, even if it seems as if it's about to come off. Let it fall off on its own. If you notice pus or redness at the base, or if your baby seems to feel pain each time you touch the cord area, let your pediatrician know, as the area may be infected. Most cords dry up and fall off without infection.

Traditional cord care recommendations used to involve gently cleaning the base of the stump once or twice a day with rubbing alcohol. But in recent years, some evidence has emerged to suggest that this once-standard practice does not make the cord dry up and fall off more quickly than if it's simply left to dry out on its own. Furthermore, rubbing alcohol—which was the traditional germ killer of generations past—may not work as well as other topical substances, such as the antifungal gentian violet. Shortly after the cord is cut following delivery, it may be treated with an antimicrobial dye. This one-time application usually is enough to prevent infection.

myth
Nighttime/daytime bathing is best/worst.

reality
Choose what works for you and your baby.

the facts

Some parents like night bathing because they feel that it's a nice way to wind down a baby's busy day, and that the routine relaxes him before bedtime. Other parents prefer morning or daytime baths, which can be a great outlet for an older baby's playful energy. The choice is yours—and your baby's.

After maternity leave, many working parents prefer the night bath, because they are unable to spend this special time with baby during the day. And sometimes a warm bath before bed can calm a fussy or lively baby. (On the other hand, a joyful splash in a toy-filled tub can rev a baby up!) If you choose a daytime routine, you can do it after a feeding and before a nap, and it can serve the same purpose of relaxing a baby before sleep. Or you can do it after a nap and a feeding as a fun way to wake up and play. If you live in a climate with cold winters, where the nighttime temperatures are markedly chillier, then perhaps everyone will be more comfortable with a daytime bath; but if you keep your bathroom and baby's bedroom warm, it shouldn't matter.

Consider your schedule, your baby's age and temperament (perhaps you'll change your routine when your baby graduates from the infant tub to a full-size tub), and the practicalities of night versus day within your household. Medically speaking, there's no right or wrong time of the day for bathing.

Should you treat cradle cap?

Some babies are born with lots of hair, and some are as bald as their great-grandfathers, but all newborns can get a common scalp condition called "cradle cap" (or neonatal seborrheic dermatitis). This yellowish, patchy-looking crust occurs on the scalp as new skin cells replace old ones, and at such a rapid rate that the old skin cells simply form a buildup that gradually flakes off.

As with many childhood conditions, this is one of those things that may bother you more than it bothers your baby. There is no pain or itching associated with normal cradle cap; the condition will clear up without any intervention. However, if you would like to treat it, you can do so by washing your baby's hair daily with a mild baby shampoo; while the scalp is wet, gently rub it with a soft-bristle brush or washcloth to remove the scales and then rinse. Or, before a shampoo, you may apply a bit of mineral or olive oil onto the scalp, wait a moment for the crust to soften, and then gently rub it with a washcloth or a soft brush to remove. The scales will be washed out of the hair when you rinse it. If the condition seems especially stubborn or severe, ask your pediatrician about other treatments.

myth

It's okay to leave an older baby in the tub for a moment if you use a bath seat or ring.

reality

A baby should never be more than an arm's length away from you during bath time.

the facts

Once your baby can sit upright, between four and seven months, you can think about moving bath time into the big tub. Some parents simply move the baby tub, provided it's large enough for an older baby, directly into the regular bathtub. (This works if you have one of the larger, plain baby tubs, not a tiny reclining seat with lots of built-in features.) Others opt for special baby bath seats or tub rings, which attach with suction to the bottom of the tub or with a clamp that fits over the side of the regular tub. Avoid older-model bath seats or rings with large leg openings. Even while attended, babies have managed to topple over, or to slip under the leg openings or rings, and go underwater. (Some safety advocates warn that suction cups, unless they are exceedingly strong, aren't safe at all, since there's always a chance that they'll come unstuck.)

The bath seats and rings on the market today are designed for safety, but even if you're confident that the device holds your baby securely, *never leave your baby unattended in the tub, or with anyone other than another adult as a supervisor.* Most accidental drowning happens when a baby is either left alone or is being watched by an older child, who may be old enough to be on his own in the tub but who may not be observant, quick, or strong enough to rescue a baby in distress. Even if you only have a few inches of water in the tub, that's enough to cause accidental drowning. Keep a dry towel handy to wrap your child in if you must answer the door or phone, because you'll *always* take your baby with you when you leave the bathroom.

There is a wide array of baby-friendly tubs and gizmos on the market today—including inflatable bathtubs, which can come in handy if you're overnighting at Grandma's. But some parents forgo all the extra gear and simply get right into the tub with their babies! If this appeals to you, it's cheap, it's fun, and it's loads easier on your back than hunching over a tub. (Never get out of the tub without handing your baby off to another person first, or putting your baby down on a thick towel next to the tub before you get out. Should you slip and fall, you don't want to have the baby in your arms.)

myth

After or between baths, remove normal earwax buildup with cotton swabs.

reality

It is unnecessary and potentially quite dangerous to insert anything into the ear canal.

the facts

It may not be pretty to look at, but earwax, for the most part, is harmless, and in fact is often beneficial. Its oily makeup provides a protective barrier against water in the ear canal, and it contains beneficial antifungal and antibacterial properties. It doesn't prevent your baby or child from hearing properly (unless it builds up to unusually excessive levels and causes a blockage), and normal earwax discharge is not a sign of illness or infection.

It can be extremely dangerous to insert anything into an ear (that goes for your own ears), because it's quite easy to puncture the eardrum, especially in a baby who wiggles or a young child who won't keep still. Because the canal near the eardrum is also quite sensitive, it is uncomfortable or even painful for some children. Furthermore, you may actually push the earwax back into the ear canal if you fiddle with it—thus packing it in, which can then cause a real blockage. It's safe to gently clean visible earwax *outside* of the ear canal with a washcloth or cotton swab, but do not put your finger, a cotton swab, or anything else directly into the ear. The normal wax buildup comes out on its own, eventually, and its removal should not be considered a part of a regular bathing or hygiene routine. Leave the job of removal, if it's deemed medically necessary by a doctor, to your pediatrician, or ask her to show you how to use a bulb syringe to remove the wax from time to time, or how to use an over-the-counter earwax softener.

Should you use talcum powder, cornstarch, or nothing at all?

Powdering after each diaper change is not advisable (see page 102), because talc and other powders can irritate a baby's respiratory system, nor is it necessary, given the absorbency of most diapers. But what about after bath time? Are all powders created equal, or is talc the real villain? And does any kind of powder have a place in the nursery or medicine cabinet?

Because powders are easily inhaled into the lungs, where they can cause breathing difficulties and even respiratory damage, the American Academy of Pediatrics advises against their routine usage. Talcum powder, in particular, is composed of very tiny particles that are among the most easily inhaled, and should not be used on babies and children. Cornstarch particles are larger and coarser (and not as easily airborne as the lighter talc), which is why cornstarch-based powders are popular in the baby products aisle. These products are often marketed as healthy, "all-natural" alternatives to talc. However, despite the larger particle size, cornstarch can also be accidentally inhaled like talc and has been linked to serious respiratory problems, so use caution with cornstarch-based powders. Never apply powder directly onto an oozing or weeping rash, such as severe diaper rash, poison ivy, or other forms of dermatitis.

If you love the scent of baby-fresh powder, and if your pediatrician agrees that a light dusting with talc-free powder after bath time is generally safe, sprinkle the powder in your hand, away from a baby's face, and then apply gently. Avoid creating a "cloud" of powder that your baby can inhale, no matter how safe the label says it is.

Finally, nontalc powders do have their uses. Cornstarch-based powders can be effective in treating heat rash and other mild rashes, and can keep baby's skin dry, cool, and comfortable if you live in a humid, warm climate.

Baby Clothes 101
Dressing your baby

myth
You should wash your newborn's clothing in special detergent.

reality
You can use regular detergent in most cases.

the facts
Unless your baby has highly sensitive skin, atopic dermatitis, or allergies, you can wash his clothing (with the exception of cloth diapers, which should always be washed separately) with regular laundry detergent, and with the rest of your family's laundry. You may want to wash one item of clothing in regular laundry detergent and see if it causes any reaction, before you do all the garments this way. (As mentioned earlier, some harsh detergents can worsen normal skin conditions, like baby acne.) Some families prefer—not just for baby's skin but for their own comfort—fragrance-free

detergents and fabric softeners, which can be milder on the skin than scented products.

If this is your first baby and you've received lots of new clothing, wash it before baby wears it to remove excessive sizing agents, dyes, and other substances that may irritate the skin. Consider the manufacturing and shipping process for clothing: Before it gets to you, the fabric comes into contact with many elements and many pairs of hands, and then sits in a store or a warehouse, where it is handled even more. While it may not look dirty, new baby clothing should be laundered before being worn.

myth
Dress your newborn very warmly.

reality
Dress your newborn practically.

the facts

Your mother insists the new baby should have a heavier blanket in the stroller, and a hat on her head, even though it's a gorgeous summer day in the low 80s. "But she'll catch a chill! She's just a tiny thing!" your mom says as you prepare to leave for your walk, following you out the door with a tiny crocheted sweater. Your mom's heart is in the right place, and she is partially correct: Newborns *should* be dressed warmly, but if it's warm outside (over 75 degrees), you can leave the wool at home.

Generally, newborns should wear one layer more than what you're wearing. Let's say it's a mild day, and you're wearing jeans and a short-sleeved shirt, no sweater. Besides a diaper and an undershirt, you'll want to put your baby in a sleeper or a daytime outfit, socks or booties, and for that "one more layer" a lightweight receiving blanket. (A premature baby may need additional layers because such infants may still have difficulty regulating their body temperature.) You can add a cotton hat, especially if this is in the early days. Newborns dislike cold and drafts, and if the weather is warm outside, be aware of the lowered temperature inside due to air-conditioning. If the baby is outside in hot weather, then a single layer of clothing may be appropriate. If it's cold, break out the heavier items and keep her head covered. Use common sense, as well as the thermometer, as your guide.

myth

Newborns and infants should wear shoes to protect their tiny feet.

reality

Lose the shoes.

the facts

Barefoot (or nearly) is best! For newborns, those tiny toes should usually be covered with socks or warm booties, especially if you're heading outside, and you'll always want to keep something on the feet when the temperature drops. But actual shoes are unnecessary and possibly detrimental, especially for young babies for whom walking is a still-distant milestone. Even prewalkers need to stretch their feet and flex their arches, and shoes that confine growing feet inhibit these actions. (Also, like shoes, tight, too-small socks and footed pajamas that restrict normal movement not only will be uncomfortable but can affect growth, if worn frequently and regularly.)

Indoors, it's best to let new walkers go barefoot so that they can strengthen their toe gripping, develop balance, and build necessary muscles in the feet, ankles, and legs. If it's winter and your house is chilly (or your floors are dirty!) you can find socks with skid-proof soles to prevent slipping, or soft-soled booties that don't restrict the feet.

Shoes on babies who can't yet walk may finish off an outfit for that family photo session, but snap the pictures and take the shoes off when you're done. Shoes on toddlers are usually necessary for going outside (though a shoeless walk in the grass or on a beach is a thrill), keeping the feet warm, or offering traction on smooth surfaces, but barefoot walking indoors increases agility and balance and should be encouraged. (For more myths related to walking, see chapter 6.)

Safe in the Sunshine
Protecting your baby's skin

myth
Sunscreen should not be used on infants younger than six months.

reality
You can—and should—apply sunscreen on babies' skin, with care. Older babies, toddlers, and preschoolers should wear sunscreen for outdoor activities.

the facts
In previous generations, pediatricians suggested that mothers give babies regular sunbaths and park their carriages or strollers in direct sunlight, to promote "healthy" color and increase vitamin D production. (See pages 34–37 for more on vitamin D.) We now know, of course, that sun damage is also an unwanted side effect, and it doesn't just

cause wrinkles; it causes skin cancer. But is it safe to put chemical-based sunscreens on an infant's delicate skin? Sunscreens frequently carry this caution: "Not for use on infants less than six months of age." Does that mean all such products are off-limits?

The AAP has changed its recommendation against the use of sunscreens on babies younger than six months, and now advises their use if unprotected sun exposure is unavoidable, especially if sunburn is a danger. However, before you reach for the sunscreen, cover any exposed skin, such as arms and legs, with comfortable, loose-fitting clothing (long pants and sleeves in lightweight fabrics, or a light blanket), and add a hat with a wide brim to keep sun off the face. When using sunscreen, apply it carefully to small areas of the body such as the face or back of hands. The AAP also recommends sunglasses for children of all ages to protect their eyes. If long sleeves and pants are impractical because you're taking your baby into an outdoor pool, you should apply sunscreen on areas that will be exposed.

For babies younger than 6 months, use sunscreen on small areas of the body, such as the face and the backs of the hands, if protective clothing and shade are not available.

Read labels and choose a sunscreen that says "broad-spectrum"; this means it will screen out both forms of ultraviolet light, UVA and UVB rays. Consider sunscreens formulated especially for babies, as they may be better for potentially sensitive skin. Children's sunscreens generally have higher SPFs. The SPF, or sun protection factor, indicates how long the skin can be exposed to the sun before it burns, although these measurements aren't exact—and you certainly don't want to test the effectiveness of a particular SPF on your own skin, much less a child's. If you want to buy a bottle of sunscreen the whole family can use, pick one with an SPF of at least 15. Studies have shown that there isn't much difference between a sunscreen with an SPF of

15 to 30 and one that is 30 and higher. The AAP recommends that parents choose a product with zinc oxide or titanium dioxide for sensitive areas of the body, such as the nose, cheeks, tops of the ears, and shoulders.

Older babies, toddlers, and preschoolers should wear sunscreen for outdoor activities—not just a trip to the swimming pool (where water-resistant sunscreen is the best choice). If your child is in a summer program where playground time and water play happen under sunny skies, always apply sunscreen and pack additional supplies to be reapplied as needed—every two hours, according to AAP recommendations. Many sunscreens are effective only if they are applied 15 to 30 minutes prior to the skin's exposure to the sun, as they need to be absorbed, so you'll want to read product instructions. You can now purchase sunscreen that dries clear but comes out of the bottle in colors like purple or pink, so that you can verify that coverage is even (and perhaps the bright "body paint" will distract a squirming two-year-old who can't wait to hit the water). There are also sunscreen sprays, mists, roll-ons, and wipes, all designed to make kid-friendly sun protection a little easier for parents (and after they've used it on the kids, they should remember to put it on themselves).

Don't get burned by these facts (this goes for grown-up skin, too).

Clothing alone may not always protect the skin from the sun. The sun's rays can penetrate some clothing. (Some studies estimate that the SPF factor—the sun protection factor—of a regular cotton T-shirt is about 7, which is considered to be minimal by skin cancer experts.) Some parents prefer children's swimsuits and other outdoor clothing made from special fabrics that block the sun's rays, known as UPF fabric (ultraviolet protection factor). For babies and children, look for a UPF of 40 or higher.

Sunlight can cause skin cancer even if the skin never gets burned. You should avoid sunburn, but even if a serious sunburn—complete with blisters and subsequent peeling—never occurs, skin cancer is always a risk of prolonged exposure.

Sunscreen is important, but it won't prevent all long-term skin damage. It would be nice if simply using sunscreen daily prevented all skin damage, but sunscreen isn't a magic bullet. Use it regularly, but add common sense to your routine and be aware of how much time is spent in the sun.

Sunburn happens year-round, even in snowy weather (even if it's cloudy). If you're not a skier but you wonder why they always have those funny tan lines around their eyes in January, it's because the snow can reflect up to 85 percent of the sun's rays (and the sun is so powerful that it can burn unprotected skin even on an overcast day). Not wearing sunscreen in the snow is like going to the beach without so much as a hat. Protect your child's skin, and yours, from the sun four seasons a year.

myth
If your child has eczema, don't allow him to go in the sun or go swimming.

reality
Most children with eczema can enjoy summer fun, including water play.

the facts

Eczema, which can develop in infancy or not appear until later in childhood or adolescence, is a general term for a noncontagious skin condition that affects about 10 percent of all babies and children. Its main symptom is itchy, dry skin, often on the face or trunk, but also on the hands, behind the knees, in the bend of the elbows, and elsewhere. It may start out with tiny bumps, which naturally become scaly, red, and irritated the more a child scratches the skin. It is very difficult for a baby or young child not to scratch, and if he is rubbing the skin raw or breaking the skin with his fingernails, it will definitely make the situation more uncomfortable.

If your child has recurring patches of dry, irritated skin that you suspect may be eczema, point them out to your pediatrician and consult on the best treatment, which may include steroid creams or antihistamines, or may initially involve some simple preventive measures, such as limiting or changing bathing patterns (see the box on pages 97–98), using lukewarm, not hot, water, and using moisturizers to keep the skin from drying out. While there is not a cure for eczema, it can be managed successfully.

Winter can be tough for eczema sufferers, since cold weather and overheated homes or preschools can aggravate dry skin. But when summer rolls around, is it okay to let a child with eczema swim? Some eczema sufferers are not bothered by chlorinated water or ocean water (freshwater usually presents no problem), but both can dry the skin out. Make sure to rinse off pool or saltwater completely, and follow up with a moisturizer. It's okay to expose eczema to the sun (though a sunscreen is essential), but high temperatures combined with perspiration can cause itching and flare-ups.

Many children (including 60 percent of babies who have it) outgrow eczema, though they may have sensitive skin as adults and can also be at risk for developing asthma and allergies, as there seems to be a link between eczema and asthma and allergies. More than half of all children with eczema later develop hay fever allergies or asthma.

Eczema's causes are sometimes genetic or difficult to pinpoint, so the best tactic is to focus on treatment and prevention rather than cause. Your pediatrician can help you identify potential skin irritants that serve as "itch triggers" such as a synthetic fiber or fabric, certain metals, chemical substances (perhaps in a lotion or soap), or known trigger foods. Upper respiratory infections, temperature changes, animal dander/saliva, and feeling hot or sweating can also trigger eczema. It is important to note that children (and adults) can differ considerably with respect to their specific eczema triggers, and these can sometimes be difficult to identify.

To bathe or not to bathe? With eczema, that is the question.

If your child has eczema, perhaps you've received conflicting advice on whether or not to limit baths. "Avoid excess bathing." "A daily bath can be hydrating." So, which advice is correct? It turns out both approaches have some merit. With eczema, bathing can be part of the solution or part of the problem, depending on how it is done. The American Academy of Dermatology offers a variety of bathing suggestions and preventive measures that may take the edge, if not the itch, off your child's eczema symptoms.

Check the water temperature. Obviously you would never use hot water to bathe a child for safety reasons, but very warm water will dry the skin out and exacerbate eczema. Use lukewarm water for bathing and cool water for hand-washing.

Second-guess the soap. Using soap isn't always necessary at every bath, particularly if a child isn't dirty or sweaty. The diaper area, hands, feet, armpits, and neck (where milk can collect) may require mild soap, but sometimes water is sufficient. Use care on the delicate facial skin, which may not need any soaping. Choose a gentle, perfume-free soap or cleanser formulated specifically for sensitive skin. If the product causes any irritation, stop using it immediately.

No rub-a-dub-dub allowed. Do not rub or scrub the skin, and avoid washcloths and sponges. Yes, those tiny baby washcloths are especially soft, but they still create friction against the skin. Use your hands to lather up or apply cleanser. To dry the skin, pat it with a soft towel and avoid rubbing.

Follow up with moisturizers. After bathing, use a form of moisturizer immediately. If you apply it when your child's skin is still damp after patting dry, you can lock in its hydrating effects. Choose an oil-based product, as it will hydrate and protect the skin more effectively than most water-containing creams, particularly in the winter months or whenever humidity is low. As with soap and cleansers, choose a fragrance-free product designed for sensitive skin; if the product causes a reaction and the eczema worsens, discontinue its use.

Limit bath time, not necessarily bath frequency. Depending on your child's individual condition, daily baths may actually help and not worsen eczema, if done properly. Baths are relaxing, and they can remove the crusting that eczema causes. However, a sponge or tub-bath should last only between five and ten minutes.

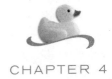

diapers, disposable training pants, and potties

the truth about diapering and toilet training

Have you noticed how all your friends and relatives seem to have lots of advice on how to change a diaper ("Why are you buying *that* brand?"), but no one actually wants to do it for you? Same with toilet training—they're all ready with a tip, but would much prefer that your child be neither seen nor heard during this phase. Feeding and sleeping are among the top concerns of most parents, but I'd bet that pooping probably has a place of honor as well. (We pediatricians sometimes call it "toileting," but I doubt you will ever use that word at home, unless you are playing Scrabble.) And just when you've mastered the Squirming Diaper Change Challenge (performed on a verbal toddler, aboard a crowded airplane), it's time for the real deal: toilet training. Here are the facts on these topics, as well as the myths you can toss out along with that dirty diaper.

Diapers (and a Bit of Digestion)
Don't do anything "rash"

myth
Always use a disinfectant baby wipe and diaper cream at each diaper change.

reality
Babies have different diapering needs.

the facts
If you've got a newborn, you've already become an expert at changing diapers, which you probably are doing every two hours. You already know to keep all your supplies within arm's reach, and never to leave your baby unattended on a changing table, bed, or other diaper-changing station. But do you sometimes wonder if you're doing it right, if you're skipping a step, or doing one too many?

New parents are bombarded with diaper-related products, from wipes and wipe warmers to ointments, creams, and the diapers themselves. Of course you need the diaper, but do you really need to use a wipe and cream with each change?

Since babies, especially newborns, have extremely sensitive skin, many pediatricians suggest you use lukewarm water and cotton balls or a soft washcloth to wash and dry the skin. But wipes are definitely more convenient, especially if you're not at home. Choose unscented, alcohol-free wipes to minimize irritating your baby's skin, and switch to the warm water method if you notice any reaction to them. Most babies will be okay with wipes (and remember never to rub—just wipe). You may wonder if you must use a wipe (or water) if your baby has only urinated and not had a bowel movement. He may appear to be clean and dry because today's disposable diapers are so absorbent. However, because urine can irritate the skin, it's a good idea to gently clean during most diaper changes.

As for ointments, creams, and lotions designed to prevent or treat diaper rash, all babies will get diaper rash at some point, and a thin film of petroleum jelly or other over-the-counter diaper rash preparation recommended by your pediatrician will speed up healing. Diaper rash is most common between the ages of eight and ten months. It often occurs with the introduction of solid foods, and is less common in breast-fed babies. If it seems that your baby is particularly prone to diaper rash, the regular, preventive use of an ointment is recommended. If you're the parent of the lucky baby who is almost always rash-free, then it's fine to skip the application on clear skin, but reach for the ointment as soon as the rash begins to appear.

In some cases, your baby may require an over-the-counter antifungal ointment such as clotrimazole (Lotrimin) or a prescription antifungal such as Mycostatin (Nystatin) to treat a monilial diaper rash (one caused by a yeast infection), which generally consists of fine bumps and affects the thighs, genitals, femoral creases (where the thigh meets the trunk), and lower abdomen (less so the buttocks). One feature that is helpful in distinguishing yeast rashes from contact or irritant cases is the presence of the rash in the folds and creases of the thighs and buttocks. Contact rashes tend to involve only the exposed areas, sparing the creases and folds. Such yeast rashes are seen more commonly in babies taking an antibiotic for another reason.

myth

Sprinkle baby powder on your newborn after you change her.

reality

There's no need to use powder on your baby's skin.

the facts

Baby powder manufacturers would like you to believe that their product should be an essential part of your baby's day-to-day care as a diaper-rash preventive. However, the use of powder is not necessary, nor is it advisable, because of its potential to irritate the respiratory passages. Cornstarch, often promoted as a healthy and inexpensive alternative, is also a bad idea, since it can trigger the growth of fungi. (For more on why to skip the baby powder, see pages 88–89.)

myth

Buy the best disposal diapers, wipes, and ointment on the market.

reality

Not all diapers, wipes, and ointment are created equal—but they're pretty close.

the facts

Even before you bring your newborn home, "they" find you—the makers of diapers, wipes, formula, food, medications, toys, and those "Mommy and me" classes. It starts with a postcard or an e-mail, and if you respond to their offers, you'll be guaranteed a steady supply of correspondence until your child hits puberty. Because they want your business for years to come, these companies try to convince you that nothing matters more than the safety and comfort of your child and that their diaper or lotion or potion will make the difference. While your baby may be your priority, you don't need to bust into his piggy bank to meet his day-to-day needs, especially when it comes to diapers.

In recent years, many large drugstore and supermarket chains, as well as price clubs and baby "big box" stores, have started manufacturing and selling their own store brands of baby-care items. These products, including disposable diapers, wipes, and diaper rash preparations, are often very close in quality to name-brand items. If you're cost-conscious and not brand-loyal, check out store brands. Compare quality, read labels, and experiment with different products. Unless your pediatrician has specifically prescribed or recommended a certain product because your child has special needs, you may be able to save significantly during the diaper years. (As the parent of three teenagers, I suggest you put off brand-consciousness in your child for as long as possible.)

myth

Never leave an infant in a wet or soiled diaper for more than twenty minutes.

reality

It's best to change diapers as soon as they're wet or soiled, but there's no twenty-minute rule.

the facts

Of course you'll want to change your baby's diaper as soon as you realize it's wet, and especially if it's soiled with a BM, and her usually sweet baby scent isn't so sweet. But this isn't always going to be possible. She may not wake up at night when she's wet, and you'll sleep through it, too. You may be in transit, behind the wheel of a car or on an airplane about to land. You may find yourself away from home without a spare diaper (and you won't make that mistake again). Her great-aunt Mary, who is baby-sitting for the afternoon, may not realize she needs a change if she doesn't fuss. For whatever reason, twenty minutes goes by, then thirty, then one whole hour. Will your baby turn into a miserable mass of diaper rash? If she's not fussing, has she gotten too comfortable with a soiled diaper, ruining her chances for successful toilet training? Will you get a citation by the Diaper Police?

If you are using an absorbent disposable diaper (and assuming you're not experiencing a Leak Disaster or a Change-My-Diaper-Now meltdown), then don't panic if you can't make a change right away. Cloth diapers may present more of a challenge, depending on what or who your baby is sitting on. Get to it as soon as you reasonably can, and keep in mind that while leaving a wet diaper on your baby won't be the reason she quits speaking to you when she hits fourteen, it does increase her chance of diaper rash. (Newborns, who can go through ten diapers a day, should be changed about every two hours; you'll find that you'll do this automatically because of their frequent feedings.)

Should you wake a sleeping baby to change a wet diaper? Most experienced parents will answer with a resounding "No!" unless your baby has a diaper rash problem or is a very sound sleeper. If it's a normal nap and a "normal" diaper (just wet, not a blow-out), give the baby and the diaper a rest until the nap is over.

You may even master the art of changing a diaper without waking your child. Some parents recommend a diaper check a few hours after they put the baby to sleep, right before they go to bed themselves. This is a risky proposition, however, if you have a baby who is difficult to put down for the night, and who will wake up during a check and change. If you need to remedy a wet diaper and can do so without disturbing the baby, then learn to do a quick, quiet change. The benefit is that grown-ups sleep easier knowing that baby's dry; and baby won't wake up wet and whimpering in the wee hours needing to be changed, or wake up soaked through the next morning.

myth
Cloth diapers/disposable diapers cause diaper rash.

reality
Moisture—whether present in a cloth or a disposable diaper—is to blame, so don't make a choice of cloth or disposable based on diaper rash potential.

the facts
Despite the 80 percent market share of disposable diapers, cloth diapers—the only option until the invention of disposables by a forward-thinking mother in the late 1940s—are still a popular alternative among some parents; but they get a bad rap as a cause for diaper rash.

Disposable diapers also have their detractors, since they can be left on longer and therefore contribute to the problem. However, it's not necessarily the material of the diaper itself that's causing the skin irritation. It's the fact that no matter whether you use cloth or disposable, the skin gets wet; friction may occur; and urine and stool contain substances that naturally irritate the skin over a period of time. While absorbent disposal diapers do keep moisture away from the skin more effectively than cloth, if they are left on for too long they will cause diaper rash. A baby in a more frequently changed cloth diaper may avoid diaper rash entirely. The likelihood of one or the other type of diaper causing a rash depends largely on a caregiver's approach to diapering.

Both cloth and disposable diaper advocates have staked out environmental positions to support their choices. Cloth users say that disposables contribute up to 2 percent of all municipal waste. Disposable users say that since cloth diapers involve laundering, as well as rinsing or flushing waste, they use up energy and water, and cause air and water pollution. However, there is some research to support the claim that disposables are worse for the environment than cloth, since discharging treated water (from laundering or flushing waste) into the water supply where it is recycled may have less environmental impact than placing solid waste into landfills.

Either way, it's your choice, and it's packed with variety. For disposables, you can choose from inexpensive store brands to premium brands, or even "green" disposables that strive to be more environmentally friendly. Disposables are generally more absorbent than cloth and therefore are particularly useful at bedtime or during other long stretches of time (such as car travel). Cloth diapers have come a long way: some have flushable liners (which eliminate the need for rinsing out soiled diapers) and extra-thick fiberfill that increases absorbency. Cloth diapers are also available in different sizes, with snaps or elastic for better fit, and in fibers ranging from cotton to hemp. If you're worried about pricking baby with safety pins, you can use diaper tape. (For more on treating diaper rash, see pages 100–102.)

myth

A baby or child who doesn't have a bowel movement every day is likely to be constipated.

reality

A baby or child can have a BM after each meal or go for days without one and still be "normal."

the facts

Depending on whether they are breast- or formula-fed, babies have very different patterns when it comes to BMs. Breast-fed newborns often stool after every feeding; formula-fed newborns do so less often, but daily. The first stools in newborns are similar, no matter how they are fed. These dark, tarry stools in the first days of life will give way to softer BMs—mustard-yellow-ish in breast-fed babies and usually tan or darker yellow in formula-fed. If your baby's stools are dry or hard, he may be dehydrated, so check with your pediatrician. As a baby grows, and certainly once he's eating solid foods, his patterns will change dramatically. Stools become much firmer (and not as pleasant as far as smell goes!), though be on the watch for hard, dry stool—again, dehydration or constipation may be an issue.

Depending on his diet, your baby or young child may not have a daily BM, which doesn't automatically signal constipation. In fact, when they reach the two-to-three-month age range, both bottle- and breast-fed babies may decrease in BMs to every three or four days, or even once a week—a significant decline from their first eight weeks of life.

As with adults, patterns will vary widely. Signs of constipation at any age include obvious straining with discomfort during a BM (see the following section; this may be harder to detect in a newborn or a preverbal infant), abdominal pain after a BM, dry and hard stools with three to four days between such BMs, blood in the stool, and soiling in between BMs. Never diagnose constipation and give your child a laxative or other medication without consulting your doctor. Laxatives (and antidiarrheals) given without a doctor's supervision can be very harmful to children. If your child is constipated, the problem can often be resolved quickly with simple dietary changes, such as adding more liquids and fiber.

myth

A baby who strains while having a BM must be constipated.

reality

Constipation is defined by hard, difficult-to-pass stools, not by the sounds your baby makes.

the facts

Even the most delicate-seeming babies and sweetest of children are capable of making big, loud, and alarming noises, such as grunting and straining during a BM, or passing gas. New parents often can't believe that such sounds are emanating from a little person, as the sounds are so adult. But babies are completely uninhibited when it comes to vocalizing during such seemingly private moments, as they are years away from learning what's socially acceptable and what is not. (Let's hope it's just years and not decades!) It's perfectly normal for a baby, toddler, or young child to grunt or otherwise sound off during a BM. But don't assume that the sound and fury mean discomfort and constipation.

It's just the sound of a kid being a kid. If you have a baby, you'll be thankful for these cues when it's time for toilet training, as they'll serve as a signal that your child is ready to use the potty. (For more on signs of constipation, see the previous myth and reality.)

My baby's BMs are green!

Depending on how old your baby is, you'll probably be treated to a range of BM colors within the first few months of life, particularly if he is breast-fed. Assuming he is otherwise healthy and that his stools are normal in consistency (no diarrhea or hard stools), there's no reason to be alarmed when you find orange, yellow, and green in his diaper. His tiny GI tract is still adjusting to the big world, and to all the things that you are eating. If you've been reading up on breast-feeding, you've undoubtedly come across the word "mustardy" to describe the color of a baby's stools. Perhaps they are green, which can happen when a breast-feeding mother consumes cow's milk products. Maybe they are yellow, possibly a reaction to a naturally occurring (and harmless) bacteria in his gut that he's learning to manage. Unless his stools are chalky white (a possible sign of liver dysfunction), bloody, or tarry black (the black may signify dried blood), you needn't worry.

On to the Potty
*The moment you've been waiting for
(and you may have to wait a while)*

myth

Your child must begin toilet training no later than eighteen to twenty-four months of age.

reality

There is no definite time frame for toilet training.

the facts

You're at a playground with your three-year-old, who is still in disposable training pants, when the mother of an eighteen-month-old proudly announces, "She's using the potty all the time. At this rate, we'll be out of diapers by her second birthday!" You want to hurl your overstuffed diaper bag into the sandbox, since your child shows absolutely no sign of wanting to use the toilet.

Now is the time to remind yourself, once again, that all children are different, and that toilet training hinges largely on a child's developmental and physical readiness, not on a specific age. You know this is the case because your child, this same one who refuses to sit on a potty, walked at ten months, while the child up the block didn't even try until fifteen months. Meanwhile your niece started to talk clearly at eighteen months, and you couldn't understand a word your daughter said until she turned two. Some children begin to lose baby teeth at age five, but others won't lose a first tooth till age seven or eight. Your son was reading by the time he finished kindergarten. His best friend didn't read until second grade. Parents are bombarded with information on what their children should be doing by certain ages, in books, in well-intended handouts from their pediatrician's office, on Web sites, and from other parents. But unless your child has genuine developmental issues (diagnosed by a clinician and not by your mother-in-law), these timetables are meant to serve as guidelines, not dates that must be adhered to. It's worth remembering this every time your child approaches another milestone in his young life, which is frequent. This is especially true with toilet training.

Children, both male and female, can show interest in toilet training before their second birthday, or as late as age three. You may be planning to enroll your child in a preschool or day care that requests all children be toilet trained or in process, though some children will be as young as two and a half. This is a common reason that some parents feel pressure to start toilet training before age two, though studies have shown that training before twenty-four months often backfires. Children who begin training before age two often take until age four or longer before they are completely trained; children who wait until age two are usually trained completely by their third birthdays.

Let your child be the guide, and look for these signs of readiness before you embark on training:

- *Your child stays dry for two to four hours and wakes up from naps dry.* This is a sign that the bladder can be controlled. Up until now, the bladder emptied more frequently. Now your child can begin to learn some control over his muscles.

- *Your child shows an interest in the toilet and the potty.* Your toddler may suddenly develop a keen interest in watching other family members use the bathroom. Let him (or her) observe—preferably with the same gender; a child may be confused if he (or she) watches a member of the opposite gender, as demonstrating works better than trying to explain it with words. If you've purchased a potty chair, let your child sit on it fully clothed and make it "his" possession, and talk about what the purpose of the potty is. Some children will drag the chair (empty, of course!) around the house and play with it, which is their way of getting comfortable with the whole notion. Some parents forgo a potty chair and use a small padded toilet seat that fits over a regular toilet. This is a good option if space is limited or if you don't want to deal with cleaning a potty, but make sure your child can get safely off and on the toilet seat. (See pages

117–118 for more about potty chairs versus toilet
seat inserts.)

■ *Your child gives you visual or verbal cues when he needs
to use the bathroom.* All that indelicate grunting he did
as a baby once alarmed you, but now when you hear
it, use it as a cue to get your child to the potty or toilet.
Teach him language for toileting and the parts of the
body involved so that he can clearly communicate his
needs to you. Make sure he is wearing clothing that
he can pull down or unfasten without tremendous
fuss. A child may also express displeasure when he
has a soiled diaper, and may tug at it or even try to
remove it himself, another sign of readiness.

■ *Your child shows an interest in wearing underpants
instead of diapers.* Some children are very proud
of their first underpants (hence the tendency to
show them off to any interested parties). This is an
important first step in getting out of diapers. If your
child is averse to underpants, don't push it. That
doesn't mean he isn't interested in potty training, and
this is when disposable training pants can come in
very handy. (These products are controversial in some
circles, but see the next myth, on page 113.)

Is it true that you can toilet train a baby less than one year of age?

A young Asian couple with an infant surprised their childless
friend by asking to use the bathroom—because their eight-
month-old baby had to go. It turns out that a Chinese grandmother, and their Chinese baby-sitter, had successfully been
training the baby to use the toilet (at least most of the time).
While the Western friend was amused, she later began to

see references to "infant potty training" and the "diaper-free" movement, with lots of enthusiastic testimonials from parents whose babies were toilet trained before they could walk.

Though the practice is rare in the United States, more than 50 percent of all babies worldwide are toilet trained before their first birthday. In parts of Asia and Africa, where disposable diapers aren't the norm, it's routine. However, despite its popularity in the rest of the world, and the growing enthusiasm for it in the United States, it's not easy to master. You must be willing to learn a very specific series of verbal and physical cues from a young baby, since the entire practice is based on being able to anticipate when an infant needs to urinate or have a BM. It also must be done consistently. Of course, some parents embrace the intensity of this kind of training because they believe it strengthens the infant/parent bond and enables the earliest form of preverbal communication. While the AAP and other medical groups caution against toilet training before a child is ready, clearly this unique method works outside the Western world, and it is gaining a tiny foothold in the United States.

myth

Don't use disposable training pants—they'll prolong toilet training.

reality

Using disposable training pants during toilet training is okay.

the facts

If you rely on disposable training pants—which are also called pull-ons—will you inadvertently extend the amount of time it takes to toilet train your child? After all, pull-ons are designed like disposable diapers, to wick moisture away from the skin, so a child may not feel wet and therefore uncomfortable. She may be missing out on a physical cue that it's time to find the bathroom.

On the other hand, pull-ons are extremely convenient for the child who refuses to lie down and be diapered (and therefore, for the adult who is doing the changing). This is especially true among older toddlers. Combine a two-and-a-half-year-old's surprising physical strength (and her ability to kick, hard) with her growing sense of independence, and you may find that it's simpler to change a wet pull-on while she's standing in front of her favorite video rather than wrestle her to the ground or lift her onto the changing table, which she outgrew last month. (The "standing" change works fine for wet-only diapers; it's more challenging if a diaper is truly a mess.) The other advantage to pull-ons is that, like underwear, they are easy for a potty-going child to pull down and pull on.

When it comes to toilet training, some parents swear by going from diapers straight to cloth training pants or "real" underwear; some may caution you on pull-ons as a surefire way to make toilet training last through pre-K. Others will tell you about the "bare bottom" toilet training method, which involves allowing your child to go diaperless for several hours a day. The idea is that when she feels the need to go in her bottomless state, once she considers the messy consequences of going where she happens to be standing or sitting, she'll search out the conveniently placed potty.

Consult your favorite sources for methods that will work in your household, and ask your pediatrician for recommendations. And with regard to pull-ons, keep in mind that the main factor that prolongs toilet training is an adult who tries to introduce the concept too early to a child who isn't ready.

myth

Boys are harder to toilet train than girls.

reality

It's not more difficult to train boys, though they may start slightly later.

the facts

There are many reasons that boys are traditionally regarded as late bloomers when it comes to toilet training. Some studies show that girls do have an ability to stay dryer for longer periods (perhaps because their bladders generally have more capacity than those of boys) and show an interest in toilet training earlier than boys. But let's look at the differences before we put boys in the "late" or "difficult" category. In one study, girls stayed dry for two hours at 26 months and boys followed at 29 months; older girls were able to stay dry during the day at 32.5 months, while boys came in at 35 months; girls showed an interest in potty training at 24 months of age, while boys expressed an interest at 26 months of age. We are talking about differences of three months or less—months or weeks, not years!

There's another factor to be taken into account, which may explain why boys get a reputation for lagging behind. In many households, it's Mom or a female caregiver who takes the lead on toilet training, despite a child's gender. Children learn about and get interested in toileting from observing adults, and if a boy has fewer opportunities to observe a member of the same sex in the bathroom than a girl, it's natural that it would take longer for these lessons—including the sometimes perplexing notion of being able to urinate while standing—to sink in. All children are different, but one thing is true regardless of gender (or sitting versus standing): a child must be ready before you start this process.

Should all boys be circumcised?

Most boys in the United States are circumcised at birth for religious, cultural, or social reasons. While there is some scientific evidence to suggest that there are medical benefits to circumcision, most major medical institutions agree that routine circumcision (the removal of the foreskin at the tip of the penis) in newborn boys is not required for good health and hygiene. In fact, despite the prevalence of this practice, no major medical organization, including the American Academy of Pediatrics (AAP), advocates routine circumcision in baby boys.

Circumcision does not prevent urinary tract infections (UTIs), although the risk may be significantly reduced. About one in a hundred uncircumcised males contract a UTI, as opposed to one in a thousand circumcised males. The risk of sexually transmitted diseases may also be slightly reduced in men who are circumcised. Penile cancer, though extremely rare in general, is almost exclusively seen in uncircumcised men. Keeping the penis clean is usually easier for circumcised males, but simple hygiene can be taught at an early age with few problems.

If circumcision is unnecessary, then why do most baby boys undergo the procedure? Again, it's largely due to religious reasons (particularly Jewish and Islamic faiths), or social and cultural traditions. Parents may want their son to look like all the other males in the family, or they may worry that he'll feel different from his peers if he is the lone uncircumcised male. These are all valid and powerful reasons.

Circumcision is quite painful for babies, though the procedure lasts only a few minutes. It should be done in the first days or weeks after birth, since it is a more complicated and therefore riskier procedure in older boys. Although some circumcisions are still done without anesthesia, the AAP recommends that doctors use pain medication to reduce a newborn's stress and discomfort. In this instance, the benefits of the medication outweigh the risks of analgesia.

Circumcision is a personal decision—not a medical one—that parents should make before a child is born. It should be performed only when you understand the advantages and risks of the procedure. As summarized by the AAP, "the decision to circumcise is one best made by parents in consultation with their pediatrician, taking into account what is in the best interest of the child, including medical, religious, cultural, and ethnic traditions."

myth

Potty chairs, not toilet seats, are the preferred option for toilet training.

reality

Both work, but your choice should depend on your child's comfort.

the facts

Most toilet training guidelines assume you have on hand a potty chair for your child. These kid-sized chairs are portable and generally safe, but they aren't the only option, nor are they the best option in some households. Many parents prefer a potty seat—a scaled-down, child-friendly toilet seat, usually padded and often decorated with favorite cartoon characters or in bright colors, that fits directly over a regular toilet seat. Urine and BMs go directly into the toilet, so there is no need for dumping out the contents of a potty and keeping it sanitary. If you live in a small house or apartment, potty seats are especially convenient since they take up almost no space. They are also convenient if you're traveling overnight and don't want to break up the toilet training routine, and they are relatively inexpensive if you want to keep one in each bathroom. However, your toddler is not tall enough to get off and on the toilet without assistance, so you'll need to help out more than you would with a potty chair, and most likely you'll want to get a step stool to make it easier for him.

There's no evidence to suggest that potty seats are somehow more effective than potty chairs, or vice versa, when it comes to toilet training. It's simply a matter of convenience and lifestyle in your household. Some children may develop a fear of (or fascination with) a flushing toilet, worrying over what happens if they fall in, or if the water overflows; if the mechanics of the toilet seem to be getting in the way of the business at hand, try the potty chair and keep in mind that a toilet (or toilet paper) obsession will eventually fade. For some parents, a combination of potty chair and potty seat works well, particularly if the house only has one bathroom, or if the bathroom is located upstairs or not close to the areas where a child spends most of his time.

myth

Bed-wetting indicates a serious emotional or physiological problem.

reality

Because of how the bladder grows in a young child, nighttime bladder control isn't fully achieved until four or five years of age, and can take years longer in some children.

the facts

Before you think there is something wrong, look at what's gone right. Your child is fully toilet trained during the day and has no problem indicating her need to use the toilet at home and at preschool; she can dress and undress herself in the bathroom and clean up after herself. She is proud of what she's achieved.

Unfortunately, nighttime continence may not be accomplished for one or two years (and sometimes longer) following daytime control. Bed-wetting is common in young children up to age four; nearly half of all children age three still wet the bed, as do approximately 20 percent of all four-year-olds. In short, nighttime bed-wetting is fairly common among preschoolers.

Looking ahead, if your child were to continue wetting up to age six, most likely her bladder would still be immature—as are the nerve pathways from pelvis to brain that signal the urge to urinate—and its capacity will eventually catch up with the rest of her growth. If the problem persists past age six, you should consult with your pediatrician to rule out medical problems such as diabetes, urinary tract infections, or structural abnormalities in the bladder (though if she isn't having wetting difficulties during the day, such conditions are unlikely). Likewise, if your child has been dry through the night for three or more months and then starts wetting the bed once again, inform your pediatrician. (Such a pattern may signal a condition known as "nocturnal enuresis." This refers to nighttime urinary accidents beyond the normal period—either school-age children [age six for girls, age seven for boys] who were never completely dry or children of any age who had previously achieved control and then regressed.)

There is a very small percentage of children for whom bed-wetting persists into adolescence and adulthood, but the probability of your child winding up in this group is small. (Protracted nocturnal enuresis does appear to have a genetic basis, as it can run in some families.)

For now, unless your preschool child has regressed after having been dry for an extended time, don't make an issue out of it and don't look too hard for a reason. Bed-wetting is normal in preschoolers.

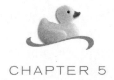

little coughs, big worries

the truth about common childhood illnesses and keeping your child healthy

Kids are cute—but did you know that 5 percent of the average preschooler's body weight is . . . *bacteria*? That's right, not sugar and spice and everything nice, but one to two pounds of good ol' bacteria. That's an astounding fact, for a few reasons. It's proof that there are lots of good bacteria out there that regulate and strengthen our immune systems and help to keep us healthy, and it's a neat fact that the older brother of your preschool darling can use to creep out his friends.

There are many myths surrounding the transmission of common childhood illnesses, with the classic common cold (caused by a virus, not by any of the bacteria freeloading on your three-year-old) leading the pack. There are also numerous myths regarding viruses and bacteria that cause some of these ailments, as well as the antibiotics, over-the-counter medications, immunizations, and home remedies we may use to prevent, treat, and manage these illnesses. None of us is immune to some of these myths (as I pointed out in the introduction, my pediatrician wife admonished one of our kids to wear a sweater or risk catching a cold), but the facts work better than chicken soup when it comes to clearing things up. (And chicken soup doesn't cure colds—see page 130.)

Colds, Coughs, and Kids
Treating them the right way

myth
Over-the-counter children's cough/cold remedies are safe, speed recovery, and achieve faster cures than letting a cold run its normal course.

reality
No child under the age of two should be given an over-the-counter cough/cold remedy.

the facts
Until late 2007, parents could shop for a wide variety of "infant" over-the-counter (OTC) remedies to treat the

common cold and cough. (In this case, manufacturers use "infant" to describe children under two.) These included pediatric versions of all four popular OTC remedies that adults regularly take: nasal decongestants, antihistamines, cough suppressants, and expectorants, often in some combination or with added ingredients such as a pain reliever or fever reducer. They had labels such as "long-acting cough/cold remedy," "multi-symptom relief," or "fever/pain relief plus cold/cough relief." All varieties formulated for children under two were taken off the drugstore shelves after conclusive evidence showed that the use of cough and cold remedies in children can do more harm than good.

Children (not just those under two) have been seriously sickened by accidental overdosing, or when given more than one type of medication (many have identical ingredients, creating a risk of overdosing; well-meaning parents may try more than one remedy to relieve more than one symptom). Side effects have included vomiting, hallucinations, breathing problems, and in a handful of cases, death. Also, studies show there is very little evidence that such medications actually work in relieving symptoms such as coughing and runny or stuffy nose. (Even in adults, the effectiveness of OTC cough medicines, in particular, is debatable.)

Based on new guidelines from such organizations as the Consumer Healthcare Products Association, the Food and Drug Administration, and the American Academy of Pediatrics (AAP), children under two years of age should not be given any "infant" OTC medications. For children between the ages of two and six, the AAP and most of its members have serious doubts about the effectiveness of OTC cough/cold drugs. Many pediatricians are against all such medications for children under six, suggesting that it's better to ride out a normal cough/cold than offer a child a possibly ineffective and unnecessary chemical substance. (See the box on page 124 for some suggestions on how to do this without OTC drugs.) If you do decide to give your older-than-two child an OTC cough/cold medication, find out where your pediatrician stands on their usage.

Treating coughs and colds safely

Now that multisymptom cough and cold remedies for children under two have been removed from drugstore shelves, many parents wonder how to treat common but aggravating cold symptoms in their babies and toddlers. There are still many safe and effective ways to help your child feel better.

Salt, suction, and gravity (for stuffy noses)   Saline (saltwater) nose drops will clear nasal passages by thinning out mucus. You can purchase drops or sprays. Do not use any that contain added medicines; ask your pediatrician to recommend a brand, or for instructions on making your own solution. Encourage your older child to blow her nose as needed. This can be a challenge, as most kids hate having their noses wiped, but it's important to keep things flowing and move the mucus out. For babies under six months, gently use a nasal suction bulb to remove mucus. At night, put a pillow under your child's mattress to elevate the head, which will encourage drainage from the sinus passages.

Water, water everywhere (for cough, congestion, and fever)   Take your congested child into a steamy bathroom to loosen phlegm and ease coughing. Steam heat clears the nasal passages and feels good. Some parents like to use cool mist room humidifiers, particularly if the air is very dry; if you do this, make sure you clean the humidifier regularly, as it can breed mold. Encourage fluid intake, particularly if your child has a fever, which depletes body fluid. Depending on your child's age, this could be breast milk, cow's milk, or water. (See page 133, on why milk does not cause increased mucus.) Small amounts of fluid, taken frequently, are easier for your congested (and tired) child to manage rather than large drinks. For older toddlers, it doesn't hurt to leave a sippy cup of water within arm's reach.

Give your honey some honey   In a recent study, researchers administered honey to children within a half hour of bedtime and found that it reduced nighttime coughing (and reduced the amount of interrupted sleep) more effectively than dextromethorphan, the cough suppressant found in many OTC remedies. Children were dosed by age (*never give honey to a baby under one year of age*—see pages 41–42), with those age two to five receiving ½ teaspoon of honey. Honey for a cough is a time-honored remedy, and this study (published in the wake of the removal of children's OTC cough/cold medications) shows that it remains an effective and inexpensive option for parents.

Single-ingredient medications (for fever and body aches)   You can use acetaminophen or ibuprofen to treat fever. (See pages 138–139 for important information on why you should not alternate these medications when treating fever.) These single-ingredient pain relievers and fever reducers are generally safe for babies over six months, but confirm dosage amounts, which depend on age and weight, with your pediatrician. Never give aspirin, which can cause Reye's syndrome, a very serious liver and brain disorder.

Sleeping it off   Don't underestimate the healing powers of sleep when it comes to recovering from a cold. You may be worried that your child is sleeping a lot during the day. This exhaustion is natural, particularly if congestion or coughing is keeping her up at night. The body needs rest, and it's important to let your child sleep. However, if your child seems lethargic or difficult to arouse, notify your pediatrician immediately.

myth

If your child has a rattling cough and yellow or green mucus, he has an upper respiratory infection and should be treated with antibiotics.

reality

These symptoms don't always signal a bacterial infection, which is what antibiotics are designed for.

the facts

Nearly all of us are aware that antibiotics have been overprescribed in recent years, resulting in their decreased effectiveness as certain strains of bacteria become drug-resistant. But when our little ones start coughing like old men and have prodigious amounts of green snot, we want them to feel better quickly, and we're often lured to the big guns, with names like amoxicillin and Biaxin. But green mucus and a cough don't signal a bacterial infection every time they occur—they are usually symptoms of the common cold, a viral infection that will not respond to bacteria-killing antibiotics. (Bacterial mucus is more likely to be green—not clear or white—but greenish mucus is not necessarily bacterial. With regard to the coughing, a common cold can trigger coughing because the upper respiratory tract is irritated by postnasal drip and any mucus that makes its way into the throat.) Antibiotics work only on bacterial infections, not viral infections, so their prescription and use on the cold virus is pointless and possibly harmful. (For information on how the cold virus is transmitted, see the next myth, "If your baby catches a cold, blame a change in the weather.")

Most babies and children will get better on their own without drugs, as adults routinely do. If your child has a cold that lingers for more than ten days, he may have a bacterial infection. But usually, he will recover as the cold runs its course. You should not hesitate to contact your pediatrician if your child has a persistent or unusually high fever, is unusually sleepy or listless, cannot feed or drink, develops a rash, or is just plain miserable.

myth
If your baby catches a cold, blame a change in the weather.

reality
Colds come from a virus, not from .exposure to cold temperatures.

the facts

Despite what your mother says, you (or your child) can't catch a cold from getting a chill because you forgot the hat and mittens, from going in and out of doors (from warmth to cold), or from going to bed with wet hair. Of course, you may *feel* a chill if you do any of those things, but that's not what makes a cold take hold. There's only one cause: a cold virus (not a bacteria), which spreads from person to person.

Your baby can get a cold if his older sibling blows his nose and then plays with the baby without washing his hands. The virus likes to enter through the nose or eyes, so if your sneezing older child merely tickles his brother's toes, it's unlikely the baby will get sick. However, if he hovers over the baby and sneezes while playing peekaboo, that will do the trick. If he touches the baby's hands, and the baby rubs his nose or eyes, get the tissues ready. If he plays with the baby's toys or uses the same cup or towel, he's leaving cold virus—which can survive on inert objects—in his path, for others to catch. (The rhinovirus—which is the most common cause of colds—can last up to three hours on the skin or on an inanimate object; some other viruses can last even longer.)

Children can average up to eight common colds per year, in part because they just aren't aware of how easy it is to spread germs that cause colds. They sneeze and cough without covering their mouths, and if they do use tissues, they may not throw them away immediately and wash their hands. They chew on pencils or toys and think nothing of sharing them. They bite a fingernail or two and then play on the family computer. So, older kids bring the virus home from school, younger ones from day care, and parents—even the most hygienic—from the workplace because sniffling, contagious colleagues don't stay home. (In the workplace or social settings, adults are more likely to pick up a cold virus from shaking an infected person's hand than from getting a kiss on the cheek. Unless the other person is a vigilant hand washer, if he sneezed into his hand or politely covered his mouth to cough into it, and then shook someone else's, he just gave them a warm greeting—and possibly enough cold virus to get them sick, too.) And colds are more common when it's cold outside, perhaps because kids (and adults) are in closer and more prolonged contact indoors. There is also evidence that the flu virus likes cold, dry winter air, which allows it to travel and remain stable.

There is one piece of advice about colds that generations of mothers have been giving, advice worth taking that the entire medical establishment stands behind when it comes to preventing the spread of the common cold: Wash your hands frequently, particularly when someone has the makings of a cold, and get your whole family into the habit.

Keeping the cold virus away

Everyone knows there is no cure for the common cold, but there is an easy, inexpensive, and effective step every man, woman, and child can take to keep colds at bay: hand-washing. Washing hands is at the very top of the list for preventing the spread of common cold viruses, as well as other germs. Unfortunately, prevention efforts can never be 100 percent effective, because a common cold is often contagious one to two days before symptoms are obvious. Nevertheless, preventive measures like handwashing dramatically reduce the spread of the virus. Here are some other everyday tips geared toward kids.

Run from the kids with runny noses. Reschedule that play date if Jimmy next door has a snotty nose, a bad cough, or a fever. It works the other way, too: Don't send your child to day care or to school if he's spreading cold germs. He'll give it to another child, and eventually it will find its way back home to your house.

Don't share. At least, don't share cold germs (as mentioned, the rhinovirus can survive for three hours). When cold-infected kids touch common items like toys, stair rails, doorknobs, faucets, computer keyboards, pencils, and markers, they leave something behind: germs, which can survive on these surfaces. Disinfect items and surfaces regularly, not just when a child is sick, with household cleaners that kill germs. You can do what pediatricians and preschools do to keep shared children's items clean, as recommended by the AAP: disinfect toys and other objects with a homemade solution of 1 tablespoon household bleach in 1 quart of water. Clean, rinse, and air-dry items that have been in contact with saliva or other bodily fluids with this bleach dilution. (The toy or item should be in contact with the solution, which should be made fresh daily, for two minutes.) Don't forget things like telephone receivers (cell phones), remotes, and towels (avoid sharing hand towels). Never share toothbrushes, drinking glasses, utensils, or other personal objects.

Teach good manners. If your child is old enough, teach her to cough or sneeze into the crook of her elbow, not into her hand, into the air, or onto another person.

If she uses a tissue, make it easy for her to throw it away on her own. Discourage her from putting fingers and hands into her mouth. This can be virtually impossible if you're dealing with a baby, and is a challenge with older kids; but the germs gain entry through the mouth, nose, and eyes.

myth
Chicken soup will clear up your child's cold.

reality
Chicken soup tastes good.

the facts

Sorry, Grandma, but your delicious chicken soup won't cure a cold. Warm soup will, however, make some cold-sufferers feel more comfortable, and maybe that's good enough for getting your little patient on the road to recovery. Unless it's spiked with the as-yet-to-be-discovered cure for the common cold, chicken soup has no unique healing powers. However, researchers have found that it does have some anti-inflammatory properties and can speed the movement of virus-containing mucus through the nasal passages (provided your child will cooperate with nose-blowing), therefore relieving congestion and shortening the amount of time that the virus is present in the nasal cavities. Warm liquids also may go down better than chilled ones for some kids, just because they feel better if a body is cold and a throat is scratchy and irritated. If your ailing child loves chicken soup and doesn't have much of an appetite for anything else, then it's a fine way to provide some nourishment as well as fluids.

myth

Herbal cold/flu remedies (like echinacea) are safe and effective treatments for your sick child.

reality

Though echinacea is usually safe, always use caution when offering children any herbal or natural remedy.

the facts

Echinacea, or purple coneflower, has become very popular in recent years in tea, capsule, or extract form as a treatment for the common cold. Other popular "natural" remedies include zinc-based formulas and the always popular vitamin C (see the following myth). Most of these remedies won't harm your child at the appropriate dosages, but there are questions as to how effective they really are. In one study aimed at kids between ages two and eleven, half of the cold-infected children were given echinacea and the others a placebo. In both groups, the colds lasted the same amount of time, and the severity of symptoms was comparable. (A small percentage of the echinacea-group kids developed a rash.)

In other words, as with many OTC cough/cold remedies, the effectiveness of echinacea in kids is unproven and you may be giving your child an unnecessary substance that could do harm, in some cases. Despite their prevalence in drugstores and health food stores, the research is still inconclusive on the many zinc- and vitamin C–based natural remedies for kids (and adults). If your child's cold worsens to the point where you need to see your pediatrician, let her know that you've given your child alternative remedies in case she prescribes any medication.

myth

Children's multivitamins and vitamin C supplements can ward off colds.

reality

Multivitamins and vitamin C can be beneficial in terms of nutrition, but they are not magic bullets when it comes to preventing colds.

the facts

Multivitamins do have a purpose, particularly when a baby or young child is not getting enough of a particular nutrient or requires extra vitamins or minerals for a certain period of growth. (See the myth on pages 34–36, for more on over-the-counter multivitamins.) But will multivitamins keep your child from catching a cold? Will extra doses of vitamin C do any good when cold and flu season rolls around?

Many OTC cold prevention products and remedies—many of them designed for babies and children—are based on high levels of zinc and vitamin C. (Vitamin C has been associated with the prevention of the common cold ever since American scientist and Nobel Prize winner Linus Pauling popularized its supposed cold-fighting properties with a best-selling book in 1970.) But study after study shows that extra amounts of vitamin C, whether taken in supplement form or in naturally occurring sources like orange juice, do not reduce the risk of catching a cold (though some cold sufferers and researchers theorize that it can slightly shorten the duration of a cold).

Most of the studies on colds and vitamin supplements have been done on adults; megadosing with vitamin C or any other vitamin can cause complications for babies and children, and is never recommended.

myth

You'll aggravate your baby's runny nose if you let him have milk or other dairy products.

reality

Milk consumption doesn't cause mucus in the nasal passages.

the facts

"If you let him have milk, you'll be wiping his nose for days," advises your mother. Many parents (and pediatricians) once believed this to be the case, but there is no evidence that milk or other dairy consumption causes additional mucus to be made. Sometimes, after you drink milk, eat ice cream, or consume yogurt, you may feel thickening secretions in your throat. This happens because your saliva (and your baby's) may thicken *temporarily* after you consume a relatively high-fat, fluid substance. But the dairy products themselves are not creating mucus in the airways or throat. If your baby has a cold, an allergy, or any other condition that is creating a runny nose, don't withhold the milk or yogurt, because dairy is not the culprit.

Fever

Keeping your cool when your child heats up

myth

A fever should never go untreated.

reality

Normal fever serves a healthy purpose.

the facts

Even though you've been told it's normal for kids to run hotter than grown-ups do when they're feverish, it's still alarming to take your child's temperature and see those rising triple digits: 101° . . . 102° . . . 103°. Shouldn't you start to lower a fever that climbs that high? It depends, but usually you should let the fever run its course. Don't fall prey to "fever phobia" (see the related box on pages 139–140). Instead, arm yourself with the facts on fever.

If your child is fighting off a bad cold or flu, or another type of viral infection, that fever is helping—not hurting. Certain viruses and bacteria thrive at normal body temperatures; a fever kicks in to fight off those invaders, and it's a signal that the body is making more white blood cells, antibodies, and other infection fighters. By reducing the fever as soon as or shortly after it begins, you're reducing its natural effectiveness in battling infection, which therefore may linger longer than if you just let the fever do its job. Fever itself is not an illness. In fact, it often acts as a remedy.

Fever: What is normal, and when to call a doctor

Depending on the age of your baby or child, "normal" temperature means different things. For instance, for a baby or child up to age three, a rectal temperature between 97°F and 100.3°F is considered normal. (Note that you will obtain different results for rectal, oral, axillary [under the arm], and tympanic [eardrum] temperatures; specify how you've obtained the temperature if you're passing information to your pediatrician, and be aware that things like earwax buildup will affect tympanic temperatures, and the intake of hot or cold beverages can skew oral readings up or down.

The AAP recommends the use of rectal thermometers for children up to age three.) Your child may be warmer or cooler depending on external conditions like the weather, how he is dressed, and whether he's been physically active. Also, body temperature tends to rise in late afternoon and early evening and then goes down again at night. Hence, there is a range of "normal" temperatures.

Here are some general guidelines on when to contact your pediatrician:

If your baby is two months or younger and has a rectal temperature of 100.4°F (38°C) or higher, contact your pediatrician immediately. This is very important, since the fever could indicate a serious illness or infection.

If your baby is three to six months and has a rectal temperature of 101°F (38.3°C) or higher, you should also notify your pediatrician.

If your child is older than six months and has a rectal temperature of 103°F (39.4°C) or higher, you may also want to notify your pediatrician.

Check with your pediatrician to confirm when you should call the office if your older baby or child has any level of fever. A pediatrician will usually have specific guidelines you can follow, depending on your child's age, whether or not she has other symptoms, and how long the fever has lasted. It's not all about the number on the thermometer. Temperature is a valuable gauge, but how your feverish child looks and feels is extremely important. If a child is running a high fever, it doesn't necessarily mean she is seriously ill (some parents think that if a fever is high, the cause must be serious, but that's not a rule of thumb). However, if that child *looks and feels* very sick, the fever is more likely to be serious. In general, your pediatrician should likely be called if your older infant or toddler has any of these additional symptoms: severe sore throat, severe earache, persistent cough, unexplained rash, listlessness, fussiness, excessive sleeping, refusal of several feedings, or repeated vomiting or diarrhea.

For babies older than three months and children up to age three, the high range for a normal rectal temperature is up to 100.4°F, as discussed; if you are using an oral digital thermometer, the high range is 99.5°F. For children over age three, the high range for a normal temperature—with an oral thermometer—is 99°F. (You can use a digital oral thermometer for children three and up.)

Some parents like tympanic digital thermometers for infants, which read the temperature of the eardrum; but they don't always give consistent readings, because of earwax buildup or poor placement (they must be placed in the exact position within the ear canal). Make sure you let your pediatrician know how you've obtained your child's temperature. Don't use mercury thermometers; they are considered dangerous because their fragile glass casing holds a highly toxic substance that you and your child should not come into contact with. Though most glass thermometers in use today do not contain mercury, glass is still not the best choice for kids.

myth
Fevers of 104°F or higher can cause brain damage.

reality
While a fever of 104° F is high, it will not cause neurological damage.

the facts
As just discussed, even if you are armed with the knowledge that it's not uncommon or harmful for a baby or child to run

a temperature that is much higher than a feverish adult's, it's still difficult not to worry, especially if a child seems truly uncomfortable. But a fever can go a few degrees beyond 104°F before a baby or young child is at risk for brain damage. As a reminder, fevers that accompany an illness are usually beneficial. They are the body's response to fighting infection. When a "bad" microorganism, such as a virus or bacteria, invades the body, the white blood cells produce a hormone (interleukin) that ultimately results in a higher body temperature, which in turn destroys the invaders.

Typically, even very high fevers that accompany infections don't cause brain damage, but high body temperatures that are caused by environmental factors—such as being confined in a closed car on a very hot day or becoming overheated in hot weather while participating in strenuous physical activity—are quite dangerous. In such extreme conditions, the body loses its natural ability to cool itself. (Occasionally, the body's failure to cool down can also be caused by an abnormal internal reaction, but the more common cause is an external factor, such as exposure to high air or water temperatures.) In such instances of heat illness, body temperatures can soar as dangerously high as 114°F and require immediate treatment.

See the box on pages 134–136 on when a fever requires a call to your pediatrician.

My toddler had a very frightening febrile seizure—isn't that extremely harmful?

Febrile seizures, a type of seizure brought on by high fever, affect 4 percent of children between the ages of infancy and age five. They cause the body to convulse and the eyes to roll back in the head, so they are scary to watch, but normally they cease within five minutes and cause no permanent damage.

Though there may be some genetic tendency toward these seizures, most children do not have a second incident. Children who have had a febrile seizure are not at greater risk for learning disabilities, developmental delays, or a diagnosis of epilepsy. (However, a child with a history of febrile seizure will require effective fever management, which parents should discuss with their pediatrician.) Inform your doctor promptly if your child has a febrile seizure, or any other type of seizure with or without fever, but don't panic about long-term effects.

myth

It's okay to alternate ibuprofen with acetaminophen when treating fever.

reality

Alternating medications is unnecessary and can pose risks for children.

the facts

It was once common practice for pediatricians to suggest to parents of feverish children that they alternate two fever reducers, ibuprofen and acetaminophen, to bring temperatures down more quickly. However, though some research suggests this can work, the consensus now among pediatricians is that it poses more risks than benefits. It's easy to make an error and confuse the sequence and dosage of medications, particularly if your child is taking any other medications. Fever reducers come in many forms, such as concentrated drops for infants, and syrups and chewable tablets for older babies and children. If you're dispensing different medicines in different forms, making a dosing mistake would be more likely.

Stick with one fever reducer (do not give ibuprofen to babies younger than six months). Ask your pediatrician if she prefers one over the other. Some may suggest ibuprofen for fevers over 103°F. Never give aspirin, or medications containing aspirin (also called "salicylate" or "acetylsalicylic acid" in some ingredient listings) to a baby or child, as it can cause Reye's syndrome, a very rare but potentially fatal illness that attacks the liver and brain.

In addition to medication, ask your pediatrician about other methods for reducing fevers, such as sponge baths with tepid water (85°F to 90°F, or 29.4°C to 32.2°C), and when they are warranted. Do not use *cold* water, since not only will this be uncomfortable for the child, it may lead to shivering, which could then raise the child's body temperature. Because fever can be very dehydrating, encourage extra fluids. Do not overdress your child or use extra blankets, and keep your child's room comfortably cool. Too many layers and too-warm air can contribute to an elevated body temperature.

Do you (or does a doctor you know) have "fever phobia"?

The ibuprofen/acetaminophen combination grew out of a desire to lower fever, as it was once thought (mistakenly) that fever was *always* dangerous, that it should be treated like an illness in and of itself, and that febrile seizures, in particular, would bring on brain damage. (See the myth on pages 133–134, "A fever should never go untreated," and the box on febrile seizures on pages 137–138.) This "fever phobia," a term coined in 1980 by pediatrician Barton Schmitt, M.D., who studied parents' misconceptions about fever, persists to this day, although we now recognize that fever serves a real purpose, as both an indicator of what is going on in the body and a defense mechanism for fighting infection. The parents in Schmitt's survey believed that even mild fevers were dangerous and could cause seizures, brain damage, and even death, and so they treated their children's fevers aggressively, with sponge baths and with alternating medications. Other common worries included the belief that if left untreated, a fever from an infection would rise unchecked (fevers from infection generally peak at 105°F or 106°F, or lower); that a high fever was caused by something serious (like an exotic virus or a rare illness); that a temperature would always drop to normal with treatment—and if it didn't and the fever couldn't be "broken," the consequences would be dire.

But parents aren't the only ones who have fueled fever phobia. It turns out that we pediatricians, as a group, have also contributed to this myth. In a survey of pediatricians' views regarding fever, most agreed that elevated body temperature was a risk that could cause brain damage or death. Though this may happen in a few extreme cases (such as when fever rises at an abnormally rapid rate), it's rare. The researchers also asked pediatricians why they continued to prescribe alternating meds, even though it posed risks. A third of the pediatricians responded that they were doing so based on recommendations from the American Academy of Pediatrics—even though the AAP has never endorsed this practice.

myth

Children with fever should not be allowed outdoors.

reality

A child with a mild fever can play indoors or out.

the facts

When children are feverish, we may assume (wrongly) that it hits them as hard as it hits us adults, and that staying in bed or on the couch and taking it easy is what will make them feel better. Generally, though, the listlessness and irritability we associate with fever doesn't hit most kids until the thermometer rises to over 101°F. In fact, a feverish child may act normal in terms of wanting to play and interact. If the weather is mild (not hot), and your child has the energy and desire to be outdoors, then a little fresh air from a walk in the stroller or a game in the backyard may be better than sitting inside (where more germs may be lingering). However, if temperatures outside are hot, it's better to keep cool indoors, since excessive heat can cause body temperature to rise (and lead to heat exhaustion).

Ear Infections and Sore Throats
"Mommy, it hurts when I swallow!"

myth

Almost all children get ear infections, which need to be treated with antibiotics.

reality

Ear infections are very common, but are manageable—not always with antibiotics.

the facts

If it seems that parents you know are always talking about their kids' ear infections, it's because this ailment is as common as the common cold, particularly among children younger than age six. Many pediatricians would agree that during the winter months, they see more patients for ear-aches and infections than for anything else. Your child is not doomed to have loads of ear infections simply because she's a child, however. While some babies, toddlers, and older children do seem more prone to acute otitis media, or middle ear infection, it can be managed, and antibiotics aren't always the answer.

Kids get more ear infections than adults because their eustachian tubes (named for the sixteenth-century anatomist Eustachius), which connect the middle ear to the back of the throat, are shorter and horizontal. Until the tubes mature and grow longer and begin to slant downward, it's easier for germs to enter them and for the tubes to become blocked (with fluid that germs like to breed in) because of poor drainage. Acute otitis media (AOM) often follows a cold or flu (unlike the cold virus, otitis media is not passed from person to person); a runny or stuffy nose can cause the eustachian tubes of one or both ears to fill with fluid, which kicks off the infection, or at the very least, painful pressure (the resulting earache).

If your child is complaining of ear pain (babies will tug at their ears) in one or both ears, has a fever, and is having trouble hearing because the tubes are blocked, an infec-tion is probably at work. (Temporary AOM-related hearing loss, which is usually mild, often goes undetected because the unaffected ear will have normal hearing.) If you notice bloody pus draining from the ear canal or a crust indicating drainage, the infection has caused the eardrum to rupture. Though this sounds gruesome, it's actually the body's way of naturally relieving the painful pressure from blocked tubes, and your child will start to feel better (the eardrum usually heals in about a week). However, you should let your doctor know if the eardrum has ruptured, as she may still want to treat the ear to prevent further damage.

So, since AOM is an infection caused by bacteria, and not a viral illness like a cold, shouldn't you leave your pediatrician's office with a prescription for antibiotics? Not always. If your child is under two, a course of antibiotics (usually, amoxicillin) is still recommended for confirmed cases of AOM, or suspected cases accompanied by severe symptoms. (For babies six months or younger, symptoms do not need to be present to suggest treatment. The "suspected cases accompanied by severe symptoms" criterion is for children between six and twenty-three months.) However, because of concerns regarding the overuse of antibiotics— creating bacteria that become more resistant to treatment— the AAP now recommends that pediatricians strictly limit their use in treating AOM for healthy children two years and older. Before reaching for their prescription pads (which many doctors feel pressured to do when an anxious parent is pleading for medication), pediatricians are urged to evaluate the severity of AOM and suggest relief for pain, the main aggravation. Antibiotics do not relieve pain within the first twenty-four hours, but OTC meds such as ibuprofen or acetaminophen do. If the condition does not improve within the next four to five days, then antibiotics can be offered. However, the AAP affirms that 80 percent of all children with AOM get better on their own, without antibiotics.

You may be worried about what will happen if your child falls into the "wait and see" group. Should it turn out that he needs a prescription, your child is unlikely to develop a serious illness if he doesn't get the antibiotics right away. If you're upset or worried that your pediatrician won't prescribe antibiotics immediately after diagnosis, ask yourself what's better for your child: (1) offering immediate pain relief— what he really needs—with an appropriate OTC drug and letting nature take its course, or (2) giving your child antibiotics he doesn't need, which may make treatment of future and more serious bacterial infections more difficult.

When you're offered a prescription you don't want (or need)

Parents of children with bacterial infections like AOM aren't the only offenders when it comes to the overuse of antibiotics. There are plenty of pediatricians who still reach for the prescription pad a little too quickly, despite recommendations from organizations such as the AAP for more judicious use of these powerful drugs.

If your child is two or older and has been diagnosed with AOM, and she is given a prescription for antibiotics, ask your pediatrician why it's necessary for her to begin a course of a drug she may not need, particularly if she does not have recurrent ear infections and has not been recently treated with an antibiotic. If she does not attend day care or preschool with other children, that's another reason to question the necessity of the drug. With regard to AOM in children over two years of age, the medical recommendations are clear: the benefits of antibiotics such as amoxicillin are generally small, especially when compared to the long-term risks of creating increasingly drug-resistant strains of bacteria that can be passed on to other children as well as adults.

myth
Swollen lymph glands are always cause for concern.

reality
Swollen glands usually have a simple explanation and are rarely cause for alarm.

the facts

Swollen glands (or nodes) in the body naturally cause parents to worry—your child didn't have these lumps and bumps the other day, and now they seem to be growing! Usually, though, normal gland swelling is a positive indicator that the body is fighting off an infection, such as a viral infection like the common cold. A cold, particularly when accompanied by a sore throat, causes the glands in the neck to swell and feel tender to the touch. The glands in other parts of the body (under the arms and in the groin area) similarly react based on the location of an infection. For instance, if your child has swollen glands in the groin only, it may be from a scraped knee. If the family cat scratched her on the right arm, the gland under the right arm may swell.

Lymph glands serve as sensitive indicators of injury and infection, but what is more important, they also are busily producing cells called "lymphocytes," which in turn produce useful antibodies that do battle with "invaders" (like the cold virus, or the bacteria from the cat).

If glands stay swollen and tender for more than three days, the swelling is present in glands throughout the body, the skin over the gland is red or purple or feels hot or causes pain when touched, or fever goes above 101°F, check with your pediatrician to rule out more serious viral or bacterial illnesses. Swollen glands can also indicate a cancerous condition, but this is extremely rare in children. Because kids have immature immune systems and get more infections than adults, they tend to experience more swelling in the glands. Usually the swelling has a nonthreatening cause and will eventually go away.

myth

You can tell if your child has strep throat just by checking for swollen lymph glands in his neck and looking at his throat.

reality

A strep test is the only sure way to confirm a diagnosis of strep throat.

the facts

As discussed, the glands in the neck will swell with a sore throat brought on by a viral illness, like the common cold. Strep throat, however, is a bacterial infection, and should be treated with antibiotics to prevent later complications. It is also uncommon in children younger than age three. The only way to distinguish with total certainty between a viral sore throat and strep is to confirm the presence of the strep bacteria through a strep test, or culture.

Your pediatrician will take a swab from your child's throat and grow the culture; if the strep germ is present, it will show up within twenty-four hours, and antibiotics can be started. Doctors also now are able to perform a much quicker version of a strep test that gives results within minutes. However, if the quick-result test is negative, the culture should be checked again within twenty-four hours to confirm that the bacteria are not present.

Just because a sore throat seems severe and a visual inspection of the throat shows redness and swelling, it doesn't mean strep; nor does an accompanying fever. A bad sore throat brought on by a viral infection can be very painful, and the postnasal drip of a cold can cause a sore throat—but this type of cold-related sore throat is not from a bacterial infection such as strep. In fact, strep throat infections do *not* include cold symptoms such as a runny nose. Usual symptoms of strep throat are fever, sore throat, difficulty swallowing (likely associated with decreased appetite), and tonsils flecked with white pus. (*Note:* Other viruses can cause symptoms that visually look like strep, especially to an untrained eye. Don't go by visual inspection alone, and don't start a course of antibiotics unless your pediatrician performs the proper test to confirm the presence of the strep bacteria.)

Call your pediatrician if your child has no cold symptoms like a runny nose, cough, or congestion, but instead has the following symptoms: a sore throat and swollen glands that last for two or three days and do not improve at any point (as opposed to a throat that is sore in the morning but painless as the day wears on), tonsils flecked with white, fever, chills, headache, vomiting, extreme fatigue, or irritability, all of which could indicate strep. Consult a pediatrician without delay if your child seems to be having difficulty breathing, or difficulty swallowing, or is drooling. In such cases, the infection may be a more serious condition known as epiglottitis, which is considered life-threatening, as it creates an obstruction of the airways.

Conjunctivitis
Don't rub, don't share, and don't panic

myth

Reddened, runny eyes indicate an infection, such as pinkeye (conjunctivitis), which is highly contagious and should be treated with antibiotics.

reality

There are many causes of pinkeye, which does not always require antibiotics.

the facts

There seems to be lots of confusion about the causes, transmission, and treatment of pinkeye in children (and adults), in part because day care centers and preschools often have varying and stringent rules on when a child with pinkeye can be allowed to return. The conjunctivae are the membranes that line the eyelids and the eye; in children, these membranes are normally clear. Conjunctivitis symptoms usually include pink or red eyes, tearing, a thicker discharge that may crust over at night, itching or irritation, or a feeling of a foreign body in the eye.

Viral conjunctivitis is often a by-product of a cold. Bacterial conjunctivitis is caused by the introduction of bacteria such as *Streptococcus* or *Haemophilus influenza*. Both viral and bacterial conjunctivitis are very contagious and can be easily spread from person to person, particularly among children in close quarters who may be sharing toys or other items and then rubbing their eyes. (Allergic conjunctivitis, which also causes redness, tearing, and itching when an allergen like dust or pollen irritates the eyes, is not contagious.) This is why day care centers and preschools prefer that if a child has conjunctivitis she be kept away from other children until symptoms improve or treatment begins. It's not just older toddlers and preschoolers who can get pinkeye. Young babies can also contract it, though we often think of it as a preschool ailment, since that is the age when children tend to bring it into the home from an outside environment. However, adults can bring it home as well.

There is no treatment for viral conjunctivitis, except to relieve the symptoms. Viral conjunctivitis will clear up within less than a week, sometimes in as little as three days. As long as the eyes are still red, the condition is still considered contagious. If your child has a cold and there is minimal drainage but lots of swelling and redness in both eyes, she more likely has viral conjunctivitis. Bacterial conjunctivitis features swelling plus a thick and constant discharge, usually yellow or green, that may affect only one eye; it may be treated with antibiotic ointment or drops, though like viral forms, it will clear up on its own *without* antibiotics.

(*Note:* A child with bacterial conjunctivitis may not have a cold, or any other symptoms of illness.)

Why prescribe antibiotics for bacterial conjunctivitis if it will clear up on its own? Isn't this just another example of overprescription of these drugs? Many pediatricians and parents would say yes. But one big problem is that some day care centers and preschools require that a child with bacterial conjunctivitis start a course of antibiotics twenty-four to forty-eight hours before she is allowed to return. On the other hand, antibiotics shorten the duration (and contagiousness) of bacterial conjunctivitis.

If you suspect your child has either form of conjunctivitis, contact your pediatrician and familiarize yourself with any day care or preschool guidelines. You can relieve the symptoms with warm compresses. Above all, be aware of the contagious nature of bacterial and viral conjunctivitis, which can spread from family member to family member. Don't share towels or blankets, change your child's pillowcases, discourage eye-rubbing, wipe down items that everyone touches (computer keyboards, doorknobs, faucets), and most important, insist on proper hand-washing for every member of your household. (Many of the preventive measures for stopping the spread of the cold virus apply to conjunctivitis. See the box on pages 128–130.)

Immunizations
Keeping kids healthy for life

myth
If your child is healthy, active, and eating well, she doesn't need to be immunized on a regular schedule.

reality

All babies and children, including those who rarely get sick, should adhere to a complete and regular immunization schedule.

the facts

There are numerous myths and misconceptions regarding immunizations, including: healthy kids don't need shots on a regular basis; they don't need vaccinations at all; it is better to be infected "naturally" by the disease; it is unsafe to give more than one immunization at a time, so it's better to space them out; vaccines cause autism or other serious complications and illnesses; and many other pieces of misinformation.

Each year, the Centers for Disease Control and Prevention (CDC) develop a carefully researched schedule of immunizations for babies, children, teens, and adults. The AAP, among other organizations, approves the schedule. (No such organization can force a parent or guardian to have a child immunized, but all fifty states require immunizations for children to attend day care and enter the school system.) Assuming your pediatrician is following these guidelines, this is where his information is coming from. (You can view the latest guidelines for yourself at http://www.cdc.gov/vaccines/recs/schedules/.) Numerous studies on the best, safest, and most effective timing for preventive immunizations are taken into account. Based on the latest findings, the CDC recommendations are updated annually (for instance, the flu vaccine age range has recently been extended).

It is vital for the health of your baby or child, as well as for the welfare of your family and for the larger community, to receive the recommended vaccinations on schedule. Through immunizations, we have managed to eradicate or greatly reduce debilitating and often deadly infectious diseases such as smallpox (eliminated), diphtheria, tetanus, whooping cough, rubella (German measles), measles, and polio. Illnesses that our grandparents and parents feared are no longer a threat. Yet, sometimes we hesitate because we worry about subjecting our children to biological agents and powerful drugs. Studies continue to show that the benefits outweigh any risks. Not only is it safe to vaccinate your child against preventable illness; it's one of the most important steps you can take to keep your child healthy for life.

Here are some of the more popular myths about immunizations.

■ *Vaccines cause autism and autism spectrum disorders, such as Asperger's.* The link between vaccines and autism is perhaps the most prevalent and frequently discussed myth regarding childhood immunizations. Many antivaccination advocates have claimed that a mercury-containing preservative in vaccinations, thimerosal, was a trigger for autism and its related disorders, such as Asperger's. Concerns were also raised about the link between the MMR (measles, mumps, rubella) vaccine and autism, particularly after a well-publicized British study, which was later discounted, made headlines.

Thimerosal was removed from all childhood vaccines (with the exception of some flu vaccine) beginning in 2001. However, the autism diagnosis rate has continued to climb. The search for a cause for autism continues, but there is no science linking any specific vaccination, or the practice in general, to autism. For more information on possible causes of the rise in autism diagnosis, see the box on pages 152–154.

■ *The DTP vaccine has been linked to Sudden Infant Death Syndrome.* The DTP vaccine was created to prevent diphtheria, tetanus, and pertussis (whooping cough), and is given in multiple doses over the course of several years, starting in infancy (the final dose is usually administered between the ages of four and six).

The vaccine was probably associated with SIDS because the first dose is administered at age two months, when SIDS risk is highest, but no medical connection has ever been established. Though it is still available, DTP has been largely superseded by the newer DTaP vaccine (recommended by the CDC), which performs the same function but with fewer common side effects like fever, soreness at the site of the injection, and irritability.

■ *Babies or older children with colds and fevers should not be immunized.* It is generally safe to immunize a baby or child with a mild illness.

Your child is riding out a run-of-the-mill cold, complete with a slight fever, and his regular pediatrician's visit happens to coincide with his sniffles. He's due for some immunizations. Should you postpone or go through with them? Though some pediatric practices may have their own policies, such as no immunizations if a child has had a fever within twenty-four hours, the AAP says that it is safe to immunize children with minor illnesses including colds, low-grade fever, cough, ear infection, runny nose, or mild diarrhea in an otherwise healthy child. Because it may be hard to reschedule your child's regular checkup, it makes sense to go to the appointment and see the doctor as scheduled. Once you are there and you explain that your child is or has recently been sick, a decision based on your child's condition and office policy can be made.

Myth or fact: Autism is skyrocketing

It's hard to miss the headlines about the rise in the rates of autism spectrum disorders (ASDs), such as autistic disorder (often referred to simply as autism, though it is an ASD) and Asperger's syndrome. The American Academy of Pediatrics now recommends that all children be screened twice by age two for ASDs. The move is part of a larger national effort to encourage early detection and intervention of these developmental disabilities, though it may have caused some alarm among parents of healthy babies and toddlers. Previously, autism was not usually diagnosed before two years of age, but research shows that early intervention can improve an affected child's development.

Vaccines do not cause autism and ASDs. The MMR vaccine and the mercury-based vaccine preservative thimerosal were thought to be the main causes by some groups, but research repeatedly has shown this is not the case. (A recent study in the state of California noted autism diagnosis rates steadily rose from 1995 to 2007, but thimerosal was largely removed from children's vaccines starting in 2001.) Yet, based on data from health professionals across the country, the rates of diagnosis are much higher, but no one knows for sure how many children have ASDs.

Autism experts are themselves uncertain if the rate of autism has indeed increased. What is unequivocally true is that there are many more children being diagnosed with an ASD. There are two main nonclinical reasons that autism diagnosis rates have increased in recent years: (1) The definition has been expanded from "autism" to "autism spectrum disorder." ASDs include Asperger's, in addition to classic autism, as well as other syndromes such as PDD-NOS (pervasive developmental disorder—not otherwise specified), Rett syndrome, and childhood disintegrative disorder. (2) The practice of "diagnostic substitution," where children are assigned a specific diagnosis so that they may qualify for certain services. These two reasons alone suggest that logically, the numbers will continue to rise, though there is not an "epidemic" at work. Even at its highest incidence, ASD is less prevalent a diagnosis than mental retardation, and it is much less prevalent than other developmental disabilities such as ADHD, learning disorders, and speech-language disorders.

There is no one medical screening test for ASD. Instead, during well-baby and well-child visits, your pediatrician will observe and ask you about your child's development and will help you understand the importance of certain developmental benchmarks for your child. If both you and another caregiver (such as a grandparent, a day care worker, or even your pediatrician) have a concern about your child's development, he should be immediately referred to a specialist for a more formal evaluation even without screening. If you have an older child who has already been diagnosed with ASD, there is a tenfold increased risk that your younger child may also have it.

Avoid getting caught up in the confusion over ASDs, and seek out solid information from reputable organizations and professionals. ASDs are very real, but there is a tremendous amount of misinformation on their causes and treatments.

Allergies and Asthma
Know the facts, breathe easier

myth
If you have respiratory allergies, your child will eventually contract them, too; if you don't, your child will never get them.

reality
Heredity plays a part in who gets allergies, but other factors also play a role.

the facts

If you're a respiratory allergy sufferer, you may be worried that your baby will have similar problems, such as hay fever. Or, if you've never had nasal allergies, you may think your child will be home free.

It is true that a child with one or two nasal allergy–prone parents may face an increased risk for being similarly allergic, but there's no surefire way to predict this during pregnancy or in early infancy. Only time will tell, and most allergies don't seem to be on a timetable as far as a child's growth goes—sometimes they can develop (and disappear) at various ages in a frustratingly random manner. (Children with two parents who have nasal allergies are in a higher-risk group; interestingly, allergy risk is more likely to be passed down from a mother, so if only a father has allergies, the risk is lower.)

Many nasal allergies, such as seasonal hay fever, are triggered by specific allergens such as pollen. But children do not inherit specific allergies; instead, particularly if both parents have allergies, they inherit a risk or tendency toward allergies. So, though you may be a hay fever sufferer, your child may not get hay fever, but he may develop a pet allergy triggered by pet dander, or perhaps a dust allergy. On the flip side, you may never have any reaction to common allergens, but your child seems to be very sensitive.

If your child is a candidate for allergies triggered by substances like pollen, pet dander, and dust because you and/or his other parent are allergic, you can't entirely prevent them from occurring, but you can certainly manage and reduce the risk by limiting his exposure to common environmental allergens. Make sure your pediatrician knows that you have a family history of respiratory allergies, and consult with him or an allergist, if one is recommended, on ways to reduce and manage risk.

Even if you and your baby's other parent have no history of allergies, be aware that they can be triggered by the allergens mentioned above, as well as by molds (indoor and outdoor), dust mites, and cockroach particles. In addition, chemical substances found in common items (like perfumes), as well as industrial chemicals and cigarette smoke, can act as airway irritants and cause respiratory problems, with or without underlying allergies. Most important, avoid exposing your baby or child to cigarette smoke, as it has been linked to disorders ranging from asthma to SIDS.

Avoid giving OTC antihistamines for respiratory allergies until you've checked with your pediatrician, and don't diagnose nasal allergies on your own. If you suspect your child has a respiratory allergy such as hay fever, which often behaves like back-to-back colds that last two to three months, it's time to schedule an appointment with his doctor. (Incidentally, the term "hay fever" has nothing to do with hay, nor does the sufferer contract a fever; a nineteenth-century British physician who gave hay fever its name observed that his sneezing and sniffling coincided with the local haying season.)

(For information on genetics and food allergies, see the myth on pages 30–31 in chapter 1, "If you have food allergies, your baby will, too.")

Kids and pet allergies: The problem isn't Fido's fur

Recently a friend whose child has pet allergies said that her mother had purchased an "allergy-free" short-haired cat and that the child would no longer be plagued with the sneezing and itchy, watery eyes that hairy pets seemed to trigger. A few weeks later, the friend reported that the child had visited his grandmother to meet the new cat, and within minutes he had his typical allergic reaction. Grandma kept her new pet, but unfortunately her grandson can't play with him. Is there such a thing as an allergy-free dog or cat, and does pet fur have anything to do with the allergy?

So far, the answer to the first question is not really—although at least one California company has produced a "hypo-allergenic cat" (the price tag for an Allerca-brand Lifestyle Pet can run as high as $30,000—for one kitten, and there is a waiting list). Because humans react to different levels and types of pet allergens, it's difficult to breed a cat so that it has no allergy-causing proteins. (The Allerca cats do not produce a glycoprotein known as Fel d 1, the allergen that affects most people with pet allergies.)

As for pet fur—it's not about the hair itself; it's about what happens when Fluffy or Fido licks his coat and then sheds the hair. The allergen is a protein located in the animal's saliva and skin (and with dogs, sometimes in the urine)—but not in the fur. Problems start when animals shed skin cells (dander) that are loaded with the allergen, or leave their allergen-coated hair on sofa cushions, carpets, bedding, and other places. The best method of minimizing exposure to pet dander and fur is to give the animal a bath regularly, at least once per week.

If you are willing to get a pet for your allergic child but aren't excited about bathing a hairy four-legged friend on a frequent basis, the best bet for now is a pet that doesn't have fur to lick or dander to leave behind (sorry, but bunnies, hamsters, little white mice, and other rodents can also have allergens). Immunotherapy (allergy shots) works for some pet allergy sufferers, well enough to make coexistence with a pet a possibility. Some children have very mild pet allergies, and controlling pet dander and exposure to protein-coated fur may be enough (our younger daughter has minor pet

allergies and no longer sleeps with our cat). See the suggestions for controlling dust mites at the end of the dust
mites myth below (pages 160–161), as some of them apply
to pet dander/fur. And there is some hope beyond hermit
crabs and goldfish tanks (and the high-tech kitten that costs
as much as your child's first car will), including a still-being-
tested vaccine for cat allergy sufferers. Nearly 90 percent of
those receiving the vaccine have found it effective in relieving
symptoms.

myth

Fragrant, flowering plants trigger your child's hay fever.

reality

It's not the pretty, perfumed flowers that make her sneeze.

the facts

It's the pollens from grasses, weeds, and trees—not from
the vase of tulips on the dining room table, or your backyard
rose bush—that are probably triggering your child's latest
bout of hay fever. But what about flowers, with their showy,
pollen-laden blossoms? Shouldn't they be avoided?

In some cases, when they are clearly causing an allergic
reaction, contact should be reduced or avoided. But the pollens on garden-variety flowers and flowering plants are very
sticky. Nature designed it that way so that birds and bees
could capture and transfer the pollen from plant to plant.
Trees, grasses, and weeds, however, are fertilized by airborne
pollen, which is much lighter and dryer than the larger, stick-
ier pollens on that rhododendron bush near the swing set.

Don't panic if your allergy-prone child picks a daisy
(unless she's running through a field of tall, weedy, pollen-
laden grasses to find it). But if your child has a history of

seasonal allergies, keep the house windows closed during pollen season, drive with the car windows up, and give her a bath and change of clothing when she comes home from nursery school or daycare, to avoid prolonged exposure to these fine particles. Pollen sticks to hair, skin, and clothing, so bathing, washing hair, and changing clothes is a good way to reduce its impact. For those who sneeze when they are presented with a heady-smelling bouquet of freesias, it's a reaction to the chemical in the perfume, not to the pollen on the blossoms.

myth

Babies and young children outgrow respiratory allergies or asthma by adolescence.

reality

Many will, but not all do.

the facts

You may encounter an assumption that allergies and asthma—which can be triggered by allergens such as pollens—are conditions that kids simply outgrow. One reason this is a common belief is that for some lucky kids, it's true. Respiratory allergies and asthma (as well as some skin and food allergies) can sometimes go away by the time a child reaches adolescence or adulthood. But more and more, the old prognosis that some doctors once gave freely, "He'll outgrow it," no longer holds true.

With regard to asthma, it's not that fewer children outgrow it these days; it's that until recently, there were no definitive studies that tracked children with asthma well into adulthood. A more complete picture of the numbers is now emerging. For instance, a Dutch and U.S. study from 1993 found that about 75 percent of childhood asthma sufferers, those with moderate-to-severe cases, did not outgrow their symptoms by their mid-twenties and still had persistent or recurring problems. Those with mild asthma did seem to outgrow it. Furthermore, for reasons that experts are still studying, childhood asthma is on the rise in the United States and other industrialized countries.

If your child has been diagnosed with asthma, or with allergies that trigger it, there is no surefire way to tell right now whether he'll outgrow it or not. If avoidable allergens like pet dander or cigarette smoke trigger hay fever now, they may continue to be a problem in the future—or not. Only time will tell. However, because allergies and asthma (for which there is no cure) affect increasing numbers of children and adults, there is continued interest in finding effective and long-term ways to manage them.

myth
There isn't much you can do if your child is allergic to dust mites, because they're everywhere.

reality
Dust mites need certain conditions to survive, which means that you can control their spread.

the facts
Don't confuse dust mites with good old dust. Dust mites are living microorganisms that thrive in moist environments. They can't survive on dry, hard surfaces like wood furniture and flooring, so the dust bunny living in the corner of the dining room is probably not causing any problems.

Unfortunately, dust mites like to make their home in places like bedding, carpeting, upholstery, and draperies.

They live off dead skin cells (human or animal, particularly cat), and the fecal residue that they leave mixes with dust and becomes airborne. That may sound like something out of a horror movie, but you don't need supernatural powers to weaken the enemy—just some ordinary household appliances and a little elbow grease.

Weekly cleaning of carpeting and upholstery with a vacuum fitted with a HEPA filter won't eradicate dust mites entirely (they exist in every home), but it will significantly reduce their numbers. Wash bedding weekly in hot water; choose washable synthetic blankets and comforters instead of wool and down, which harbor dust mites; encase mattresses and pillows in protective allergen-blocking covers as a base layer. Avoid stirring up dust when you clean; a damp rag that catches particles may be a good choice. Choose washable stuffed toys. Your pediatrician or allergist can give you more suggestions on additional everyday measures you can take to reduce dust mites.

Many parents use HEPA air cleaners in their children's bedrooms, believing that they catch and trap dust mites. However, dust mites don't fly, and their residue isn't airborne for long. HEPA air cleaners can reduce pet dander, pollen, smoke, and other allergens, but they don't kill dust mites, nor do they wipe out their allergenic residue.

myth

If your child is in day care (or when she starts preschool), she'll get sick and will get the rest of your family sick all the time.

reality

At home or not, kids get sick, but you can help them stay healthy wherever they spend their days.

the facts

You're planning to use day care while you're at work, or you're enrolling your toddler, who has been cared for at home, in preschool for the first time. "You'll all get sick more now that she's starting school," says your mother-in-law. "She'll be bringing home colds, coughs, pinkeye, and everything else kids get."

It's true that children do get sick more frequently than adults, in part because they've yet to build up immunities to many common pathogens. But of course babies and children don't realize how easy it is to spread germs that cause preventable illnesses. We teach children to share, but there are some things—like germs—that shouldn't be shared. Obviously, when you select a day care center or preschool, you'll make sure the environment is clean, but it's worth remembering a few basic rules, now that your child will be in close contact with many other children. See the guidelines on pages 128–130 ("Keeping the cold virus away"), and consider the following recommendations as well.

The first line of defense—for adults and kids—is always hand-washing. In a day care center, where diapers are changed and food is dispensed regularly, strict hand-washing protocols are a must. Many centers and preschools make liberal use of alcohol-based hand sanitizers, which eliminate many germs. Hand sanitizers shouldn't always stand in for soap and water, but often they are a practical solution.

Make sure your child is up to date on immunizations. Accredited day care centers and preschools rarely will allow your child to attend unless her immunizations are current.

If your child is old enough, teach her to cough or sneeze into the crook of her arm, rather than into her hand or the air. Teach her to throw used tissues into the garbage can.

Use common sense and keep babies and children with contagious illnesses—whether it's a diarrhea-causing stomach bug that's running rampant through your household or a

bad cold with lots of coughing and sneezing—at home until
their symptoms are under control. Consider what you would
want other parents in your position to do. Your day care
center or school may also have strict rules on when children
with certain symptoms, like fever, can return.

Soap and water or "magic soap"?

You used to need a sink, soap, and water to wash your
hands. Now, it would seem you can do it with a squirt of
liquid that comes out of a bottle or tube, or with a specially
treated wipe. Walk into any day care center or classroom
and you'll see the inevitable pump bottles of "magic soap"
ready for duty. But are these popular hand sanitizers, or
liquid antibacterial soaps with their germ-killing promises, as
good as or better than old-fashioned soap and water?

Alcohol-based hand sanitizers, which do not require rinsing, are different from antibacterial soaps. These quick-
drying, no-water-needed sanitizers are a good option when
soap and water are not available (on an airplane, in the car,
at the playground), since ethyl alcohol, their main ingredient,
is very effective at killing germs. However, they can't always
remove "kid stuff," like marker stains or more mysterious goo
that kids tend to get on their hands.

Antibacterial soaps are different. They require regular
hand-washing (that is, with water to rinse). Some of their
antibacterial claims are in dispute—they don't kill all bacteria,
and some research suggests that they may be contributing to antibiotic resistance in some bacteria—but they are
safe to use in place of regular soap.

So, should you steer your child to the sink several times
a day for regular hand-washing with a bar of soap, choose
antibacterial soaps only, or rely on hand sanitizers? Nothing

seems to work better than plain old soap and water (soap works by separating the bacteria from the skin, even if it doesn't kill it off before it sends it down the drain). Antibacterial soaps are fine to use. And alcohol-based hand sanitizers are a good alternative when you can't find soap and water. However you choose to do it, keep hands clean.

Baby Teeth
Cutting them, losing them, and keeping them healthy

myth

Teething causes diaper rash, fever, ear infections, runny noses, and other problems.

reality

While cutting teeth may be an uncomfortable experience for some babies, it does not cause the problems listed above.

the facts

Many of my colleagues who see babies between the ages of four and seven months often get questions from parents concerned that the arrival of a first tooth will mean the onset of symptoms such as diaper rash, and infections resulting in fever. Parents have worried over teething for generations— in fact, for thousands of years. The ancient Sumerians and Greeks wrote about teething and illness; early Hindu writings addressed the topic; in more modern history, eighteenth- and nineteenth-century Europeans debated whether teething and infant mortality were related (given the state of medicine and high mortality rates in the 1700s and 1800s, it's no wonder they were looking for a link). The fact is that teething is not painless (and some babies may grow irritable during this phase because of the resulting discomfort), but teething does not cause life-threatening illness.

In fact, it doesn't even cause diaper rash. It was once thought that a baby's saliva became more acidic during the teething process, and that the additional acidity somehow helped the tooth push through the gum. This acidity also showed up in the baby's urine, causing diaper rash. But research has proven that this is not the case. (See the myths in chapter 4, starting on page 100, for more on the causes, treatments, and prevention of diaper rash.) Nevertheless, this myth persists.

Teething also doesn't cause ear infections. Because the teeth and the ear canals have a common nerve center, a baby may seem to tug at his ears as if he has an earache, when in fact he may be experiencing gum discomfort. Some studies have shown that teething babies may run low-grade fevers (101°F–102°F). If he has a fever, it could be an unrelated viral or bacterial infection, and you should contact your doctor if it persists and your child seems ill, or if it goes above 102°F (see fever guidelines in the box on pages 134–136). But more likely, the fever is unrelated to teething. As for runny noses, teething does not create any additional mucus. A runny nose could be from a cold or allergy, and like an unrelated fever, it is a symptom that should be monitored separately from the teething process.

myth
Baby teeth do not need regular care until a child is four or five.

reality
Good dental health starts before baby teeth emerge.

the facts

Before your baby flashes you her first toothless grin, you can
improve her chances for good dental health.

Don't wait for her first tooth to appear. The American
Dental Association (ADA) and the AAP recommend regular cleaning of your baby's gums, to remove milk and food
residue and plaque that can damage new teeth. When your
baby is a few days old, the ADA recommends you begin gently wiping her gums with a clean gauze pad (try wrapping it
around your little finger) after each feeding. Continue this
hygiene until her first teeth emerge, they suggest, so that
your baby will get into the habit of having her teeth cleaned.
Then, switch to a soft-bristled child's toothbrush and
water, and brush in the mornings and at night. Do not use
toothpaste until your child is two years old (and then, use a
pea-size amount of non-fluoridated toothpaste, as kids don't
always remember to spit—at least when you want them
to). Flossing is important, too, though you can wait until
your child has at least two teeth that touch. Brush your
child's teeth for her, but teach her the correct technique
(let her try) so that she can learn what it feels like to use
the brush properly. Most children can brush completely
on their own by age seven, but you'll have to supervise
until then.

The ADA recommends a "smile insurance" visit to the
dentist on the first birthday, but the AAP suggests that this
is necessary only if a child is at a high risk for tooth decay.
Otherwise, she should see a dentist for a first checkup
when she is still a toddler, after all baby teeth are present
(usually around age two and a half). You don't need to seek
out a kids-only dentist, but one who regularly sees children
can make office visits easier, and will help reinforce the
correct way to brush and floss.

If you live in an area with low- or no-fluoridated tap
water, or if your family consumes nonfluoridated bottled

water, ask your pediatrician or dentist if your child should take a fluoride supplement.

myth

Damage to your child's baby teeth (cavities, chipped or cracked teeth, and so forth.) has no long-term impact on your child's dental health, since baby teeth will be replaced by permanent teeth within a few years.

reality

The overall health and appearance of permanent teeth are affected by baby teeth.

the facts

Baby teeth, also called milk teeth, serve a purpose in addition to helping your child chew his first solid foods. They are like placeholders and guides for permanent teeth. Let's say a baby tooth is lost before its regular life span, because of tooth decay or an accident. Unfortunately, the permanent tooth that is supposed to take its place isn't ready to emerge yet, so the existing teeth have a tendency to shift and fill the space. When that permanent tooth is ready to emerge, there is no room for it. Crooked, crowded teeth are the result, and a trip to the orthodontist is probably in your child's future.

Seek out a dentist if your child's baby teeth have been damaged in any way, and practice preventive measures such as regular brushing to avoid tooth decay. If your child consumes a sugary treat, brush soon after he's done; don't wait until bedtime, because the sugar—a primary cause of tooth decay, since cavities are caused by the acid produced from bacteria that thrive on sugar—is already looking for a way to make a cavity. And never allow your child to fall asleep with a bottle in his mouth, as this may lead to severe, disfiguring decay ("baby bottle syndrome").

myth
Thumb-sucking and pacifier usage cause crooked teeth.

reality
This usually doesn't happen unless the permanent teeth are in place.

the facts
Your baby loves her pacifier or her thumb (and so do you), and then someone tells you that her sucking habit will mean a lifetime of orthodontia. Thumb-sucking isn't entirely harmless, since it's an excellent way for your baby to introduce bacteria into her mouth, and it can be a hard habit to break among older children. Pacifier usage has been linked to poor breast-feeding techniques (see pages 12–13), and it can also be a challenge to get an older baby or toddler to give up the "binky." On the plus side, pacifier usage has also been linked to a reduced risk of SIDS (see page 53). It's also easier to break the pacifier habit than the thumb-sucking habit, because while you can "lose" the pacifier and choose not to replace it, a child will always find her thumb. However, while thumb-sucking and pacifier usage can go from "normal" to "problem" if they go on too long, these habits generally are not associated with crooked permanent teeth or malformation of the jaw.

If a child continues to suck her thumb regularly after the permanent teeth have emerged, there is a real chance that the positioning of the teeth will be affected, particularly the front teeth. However, most children cease pacifier usage and thumb-sucking years before the permanent teeth erupt (between the ages of six and twelve).

For now, you can let your baby comfort herself with her thumb or her pacifier, since it's unlikely they will cause her to need braces.

Tummy Troubles
from colic to stomachaches

myth

Childhood stomachaches usually stem from "nerves."

reality

Abdominal pain can be caused by many sources and should not be dismissed as "nerves."

the facts

If your three-year-old is complaining that his tummy hurts first thing in the morning, and he just started preschool, he may in fact have a touch of nervous stomach. Stress can upset your stomach—and it can upset your child's, too—but stomach pain has many causes. Usually, most stomachaches are mild and don't indicate serious illness, but it depends on your child's age, his symptoms, and how severe or persistent the pain is.

Once you can rule out colic (because your child is past this stage), the reasons could range from constipation to gas to heartburn to milk allergy to infection (a stomach "bug" with a bacterial or viral cause), as well as rarer ailments such as appendicitis (uncommon in children under age four) or intussusception, a "telescoping" of the intestine that causes painful intestinal blockage. Intussusception is also very rare, but it can occur in the first year of life. Obviously, when it comes to abdominal pain, you'll monitor young babies differently than verbal toddlers and preschoolers, who will be able to describe their symptoms.

If stomach pain is accompanied by fever, vomiting, and diarrhea, and if playmates or family members who ate the same food are experiencing the same problems, then a form of food poisoning is the likely culprit. You can't necessarily trace your child's food-borne illness to the last thing he ate; the organisms responsible for most food poisoning may not cause symptoms for several hours or even days. For instance, salmonella bacteria cause symptoms sixteen to forty-eight hours after contaminated food consumption, while *Staphylococcus aureus* (the most common cause of food poisoning) cause symptoms one to six hours after consumption. See the guidelines on page 171–172 (at the end of the myth on giving your sick child food and milk) for information on when to contact your physician if symptoms such as vomiting, fever, and diarrhea worsen. Again, most tummy troubles aren't serious or life-threatening, but if you can't pinpoint the source of the pain, and if it isn't getting any better, contact your pediatrician.

Colic: Baby's first tummy ache

No one really knows precisely why babies get colic, and why some get it and others don't seem to be bothered by it. Colic causes intestinal contractions, which are painful enough to cause long bouts of crying. In addition to crying, colic is often accompanied by gas. Colic can start at about ten days of age and can last for up to three (long) months. The word "colic" has become somewhat of a catchall for newborns and infants who cry, fuss, and are irritable. (Unfortunately, the end of many a maternity leave always seems to coincide with when a baby's colic ends!) More than one new mother has been told, "Your baby is colicky because you're so tense!" That's definitely a myth (although she may be tense because her baby is so colicky). Colic is a temporary physical condition in some newborns and infants, and it's not brought on by the psychological state of a mother. Another myth:

"A colicky baby will grow into a bad-tempered child." There is no evidence that colicky babies are "difficult" as children or are hypersensitive in any way. If you're a new parent and you suspect that your infant has colic, talk to your pediatrician about ways to alleviate this condition. (Consult your pediatrician if your baby has other symptoms besides crying, such as fever or low appetite.) And talk to veteran moms, who may have some creative ways around it, from running the vacuum cleaner, which some babies find soothing, to gently massaging a baby's tiny tummy just the right way. Mothers of colicky babies are the true mothers of invention.

myth

It is harmful to give food or milk to your child if she's suffering from diarrhea, as you'll make the symptoms worse.

reality

Don't withhold nutrition if your child is ill.

the facts

If your child has diarrhea, your first instinct may be to withhold food and milk. After all, nothing seems to be staying in her system, not even water. Of course the diarrhea may cease if she stops eating and drinking, but that's because the digestive process has been brought to a halt. More than anything, a sick child requires nourishment. Fluids, including milk, are very important, as all diarrhea carries the risk of dehydration.

If the diarrhea is mild and is not accompanied by vomiting, high fever, or lethargy, continue to offer her usual diet, including milk, even if you serve smaller but more frequent portions. If the diarrhea worsens, consult your pediatrician, who may direct you to change your child's diet depending upon the intensity of the diarrhea (be prepared to answer questions about the frequency of the diarrhea). Such changes may include switching to a bland diet of easy-to-digest foods, including bananas, rice, plain pasta, or toast, and withholding milk for a certain period of time. If your child has diarrhea and is also vomiting, your pediatrician may recommend using a commercially prepared electrolyte drink to help with hydration. (Do not ever give boiled milk to a child with diarrhea!) As your child improves, you will gradually reintroduce and increase protein foods like chicken or cheese, and reintroduce milk.

Most normal bouts of diarrhea require no medical intervention and resolve themselves within twenty-four hours. If not, check in with your pediatrician for further instructions, such as those outlined above. You should call your pediatrician if your child has very frequent diarrhea (watery bowel movements every one to two hours) or shows signs of dehydration, such as lethargy and decreased urination; if the diarrhea is bloody or is accompanied by high fever or vomiting that lasts longer than twenty-four to forty-eight hours; if your child is refusing to eat or drink; if a rash or jaundice develops; if she has a distended stomach or seems to have abdominal pain; or if vomited substances are greenish in color, or look as if they contain coffee grounds or blood.

Do home remedies halt the hiccups?

Your toddler has the hiccups. She doesn't seem to mind them, but should you try to stop them? You remember your grandmother saying something about leaning over and drinking water from the opposite side of the glass, or holding your breath, or "scaring" the hiccups away—yet, you have an eighteen-month-old, not an adventurous middle-schooler who will try anything.

The fact is, everyone hiccups—even babies in the womb are capable of hiccupping. Newborns do it, too. When the diaphragm is irritated (this can be caused by many things, such as eating too quickly and taking in too much air), the resulting contraction is a hiccup. The hiccupping baby or child isn't in distress (though a young baby may be bothered if he gets them while he's trying to feed), and most hiccupping episodes last for minutes (not hours or days—if they do, call your pediatrician). For a young baby, burping or changing positions can end the hiccups. A few sucks of water will often bring them to a halt if they don't stop on their own.

For an older child, there is proof that holding the breath for ten seconds or so can work (the idea of "scaring" the hiccups away is based on breath-holding). Some other popular remedies are folding the knees into the chest, chewing and swallowing dry bread, taking a few sips of a sugar-water solution, and gargling with water. (In our household, I swallow a teaspoon of sugar. My kids drink a glass of water while someone blocks their ear canals with their fingers.) However, many of the home remedies for curing the hiccups aren't designed for young kids (for instance, an article in the *Journal of Clinical Gastroenterology* suggests sucking on a lemon wedge soaked in Angostura bitters). Usually, harmless hiccups just go away on their own. (And hiccups are a minor irritation for parents compared to when kids learn how to make themselves burp on command!)

myth
Children cannot develop kidney stones.

reality

Unfortunately, though uncommon in children, kidney stones aren't just an adult ailment.

the facts

If you know someone who's suffered from kidney stones—rock-hard small pellets that can block the urinary tract and cause severe pain and sometimes infection—there's a good chance that person was male and between the ages of twenty and sixty, as most kidney stones are diagnosed among that group. However, women get kidney stones, and children can get them, too, though usually from a metabolic or genetic disorder (many pediatricians also point to diets high in salt and a lack of water intake as the main causes). Adults develop them when certain minerals or other substances build up and crystallize in the urine—in most cases, calcium combining with oxalate, which is found in many vegetables, fruits, and grains, although in children stones are often composed of uric acid. The resulting stones can cause great pain as they move through the kidneys and urinary tract.

Common symptoms can include blood in the urine; a need to urinate more often, accompanied by a burning sensation; or nausea and vomiting (and fever/chills if an infection is present). A child may complain of backache (in the kidney area) or burning during urination. If she has fevers or chills, it may be a urinary tract infection, such as cystitis. (Girls tend to get cystitis more frequently than boys. Bacteria can enter their bladders more easily, due to the shorter length of the female urethra—the narrow tube that leads from the bladder and discharges urine outside the body. When the urethra gets contaminated with stool, cystitis can result. If you are toilet training a girl, make sure you teach her to wipe from front to back, away from the urethra.)

If your child exhibits any of these symptoms or has discomfort associated with urination, it's probably not a kidney stone, given their rarity in children, but it may signal a bladder problem that should be evaluated without delay by a pediatrician. Again, stones are uncommon in children, but some major children's hospitals have begun focusing on this problem, since the diagnosis and treatment differs from methods used for adults. (Vanderbilt Children's Hospital in Nashville has opened a Pediatric Comprehensive Kidney Stone Clinic; Tennessee is located in what is known as the "kidney stone belt" in the United States, so nicknamed because hot summer temperatures and dehydration tend to drive up the number of kidney stone cases that doctors treat.)

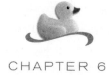

growing, growing, gone!

the truth about how your child's body and brain develop

W hen you become a parent, it seems that every well-wisher with kids tells you, "This time goes by really fast—one day they're babies and the next they're walking out the door on their own!" (You accept their warm wishes, though you secretly think, "But this colicky phase isn't going by fast enough!")

As a parent, I can tell you that it's not a myth—it can feel as if time really is racing by, if you measure it by how amazingly fast your newborn goes from delicate, tiny bundle to hearty, thriving baby to a busy preschooler who barely sits still for a cuddle. Just consider how quickly the average baby grows in terms of length. In the first year, she can grow ten inches, and in the second year, she'll add another five. No wonder your mother will say, "It looks like she grew overnight!"

At the same time a baby is growing on the outside, some fairly miraculous things are going on inside. The brain is performing some astonishing feats, as your baby begins to learn language and continues to process what she sees, hears, and feels. All the internal organs and systems that make us human are picking up steam, maturing, refining their functions, and getting ready for the road ahead.

You'll get a lot of advice and hear a lot of theories about how your child grows, and what you can do to enhance this early childhood development. As you'll see, there are some things you can't influence—Mother Nature will beat you to it—but there are also many positive steps you can take to make the most of these early years.

Noggin Power
Your child's brain

myth
Playing Mozart or other classical music for your baby will make her smarter.

reality
The "Mozart effect," which linked classical music to higher levels of intelligence, has been debunked.

the facts

If only it were that easy—play a Mozart CD for your infant and she will instantly be moved to the top of the admissions list at Harvard, or she'll at least score really well on her first-grade math test. If it sounds too simplistic, it is. But the "Mozart effect" does have a scientific basis, and in the last decade its misinterpretation has sent many parents to the classical music aisle in search of preludes and nocturnes to boost baby's brainpower.

In 1993, researchers at the University of California at Irvine discovered that college students who listened to a Mozart sonata prior to being tested on spatial relationships performed better than students who were not exposed to the music or who listened to music by another composer. A subsequent best-selling book, *The Mozart Effect* (and its sequel, *The Mozart Effect for Children*), popularized the notion that classical music was linked to higher levels of intelligence, creativity, and well-being, and spawned a line of related CDs and other products. Some childbirth educators even encouraged pregnant women to listen to classical music so that their babies would reap the neurological benefits while in the womb. The media fanned the flames, featuring stories that suggested classical music could ameliorate physical and mental disabilities.

While exposing your baby to classical—or any other—form of music can be a soothing or stimulating experience for parent and child alike, there is no evidence that listening to Mozart makes any of us more intelligent. The UC Irvine study focused on college students; the effect lasted only fifteen minutes, on average; and in a later study, researchers at Appalachian State University were unable to duplicate the effect. Even the lead researcher of the UC Irvine study said that the results were never meant to imply that classical music would make babies smarter or cure health ailments. Nevertheless the notion took hold, and the governor of at least one state, Zel Miller of Georgia, initiated a program that offered a free classical music CD to parents of newborns.

Certainly, listening to music with your baby can do no harm (unless you blast the Rolling Stones when she should be napping). Exposure to a variety of music at a young age—particularly if music is valued in your household—can be a wonderful and rewarding experience. You may find that you have a budding little vocalist on your hands, or a toe-tapping, hand-clapping performer in the making. There are many popular children's music classes available in most communities for a variety of ages, which your child may enjoy (and such classes are often an excellent first step toward introducing your baby to other babies around town). But instead of treating music as an educational tool, relax and enjoy this simple way of sharing something beautiful and uniquely human with your child.

myth
Your baby needs sophisticated toys for maximum brain stimulation.

reality
There's no evidence that a particular toy will make your baby smarter.

the facts
Black and white mobiles. "Baby Einstein" videos. Flash cards. Crib toys that play Beethoven and Bach. And high price tags. We all want to give our children special experiences and advantages, but do you need to go out and fill the trunk of the car with high-end "educational" toys? Nope. What your child—whether he's two weeks, two months, or two years old—really needs from you and his caregivers is

unconditional love, physical contact, and new experiences. (*Note:* I did not say "educational" experiences!)

The simplest activities are often the most stimulating for your infant or toddler's development—singing and talking to your child, going for walks and showing him the sights, taking him to a library (and selecting some age-appropriate books), letting him look at the funny light fixtures in your neighborhood coffee bar, allowing him to touch a variety of (safe) surfaces and textures in your home, picking him up and holding him close, just interacting. That's what your baby needs.

As he gets older and becomes more mobile, you'll find that your baby's needs (and yours) will change and he'll "get busy" at the work of play, first by himself, and then with playmates. But don't stress out if your home doesn't contain the latest and greatest in toys, games, videos, and books. It's actually easy to overstimulate a baby or young child (with your "educational outing" or game ending in tears and frustration, possibly your own). Introduce new experiences and objects gradually, and don't be surprised if he ignores that seventy-five-dollar talking puppet with the computer chip in favor of rummaging through a kitchen drawer, fingering a remote control, or playing with your wallet (which he'll wreak havoc on in more ways than one). If you're up for a trip to the toy store or someone owes you a baby gift, see the following box for some inexpensive and satisfying options.

Five baby toys that won't wreck the college fund

A kid-safe plastic mirror   She'll find her reflection (and yours) endlessly amusing. Many mirrors are designed to be attached to the slats on your baby's crib.

Small, easy-to-grasp rattles   There's a reason rattles have been popular for millennia—they're fun! Look for interesting shapes and surfaces, and sizes friendly for little hands.

Interlocking plastic rings   These rings, which conveniently hook onto strollers for easy access by your baby, have myriad uses. Babies seem to love holding them and waving them around, and of course, the rings are made to be mouthed. You can also use them to attach other small toys to your stroller. Lots of bang for your baby bucks.

One toy to consider springing for   Manhattan Toy's "Whoozit" squeaks, rattles, and doesn't roll, but it does attach to strollers, car seats, and crib slats, and has a variety of colors, sounds, and textures that your baby is sure to find stimulating. It comes in a variety of sizes and can be cleaned, which is handy because it makes an appealing teething toy. www. Manhattantoy.com.

It's the box   Yes, it's the cheapest and most kid-cliché thrill of all, but at a certain point your baby will be more interested in the box the toy came in. Just watch for sharp edges and any staples, tape, or Styrofoam "peanuts" (a possible choking hazard) that may have been used in the packaging. One more parental caution: This preference may continue for years to come!

myth
Children use only 10 percent of their brains.

reality
Children (and adults) use 100 percent of their brains.

the facts

The mistaken notion that humans, from birth through old age, use only 10 percent of their brainpower has existed for generations. It probably started with research done in the 1800s that was later misinterpreted. The myth also gets a huge boost in popular culture because psychics, "mentalists," and other believers in the paranormal suggest that most of us only use 10 percent of our brains but that they tap into the other 90 percent for their special abilities. There is no scientific basis for the 10 percent figure. Brain researchers know that even the tiniest areas of this organ affect various functions, like speech or movement. It's not true that the essential parts of the brain are concentrated in just 10 percent of its overall mass.

Your child uses her entire brain. As a parent, you can provide simple day-to-day experiences that stimulate your baby's brain development, like talking to her and offering her a variety of sensory experiences. No fancy toys are needed (see the box on pages 181–182), just some interesting everyday things to look at, some new sounds, pleasing textures, even tastes and smells that are enjoyable—and a caring, engaged adult to lead the way.

The first three years of your child's life are especially important for brain development. Researchers believe that this is the period when the brain is most primed for learning—the entire brain, not just the mythical 10 percent. That doesn't mean that if your child turns three and has not yet been exposed to the French language, chess, the violin, or a steady diet of math games, she will never learn to excel in these areas. But it does mean that you can take full advantage of these learning years and build a good foundation for the intellectual developments that are on the horizon.

Here are some simple ideas for tapping into your child's brainpower, from birth to age three, that you and your caregiver can use each day. "Brainpower" doesn't just mean intellectual development. It ties into emotional, social, and physical development as well.

- *Sing, talk, and vocalize with your baby.* If you speak a foreign language, do so with your baby (continue through the school years and watch her fluency increase—see the box on pages 185–186). Once she starts vocalizing, mimic her sounds to "talk back."

- *Hold your baby close and make frequent eye contact.* Babies love faces, particularly those of the grown-ups who love and care for them.

- *Offer interesting things to look at and begin to handle,* such as soft toys with eye-catching patterns, bright colors, and tactile qualities. Keep up with your baby's growth by rotating toys and graduating to more interesting ones.

- *By four months, start to look at picture books* with your baby. Once you get into the habit of reading (even if it's just one word per page to start, it still counts), do it daily—and do it for years to come.

- *Introduce music and rhythmic movements* (dance with your baby). In the toddler years, offer a small, kid-tested musical noisemaker, such as mini-maracas, a drum, or a tambourine.

- *Play games.* Babies and toddlers enjoy peekaboo and clapping games (like patty-cake), and preschoolers love hide-and-go-seek (even if they "hide" in front of you by closing their eyes).

- *Head outside.* Fresh air and a change of scenery stimulate the mind and the body. For new walkers, toddlers, and preschoolers, find a safe playground where they can explore and test out their increasing strengths. Free them from their strollers and let them run in the grass, pick up pebbles, stare at the bug crawling on the sidewalk, or collect leaves or acorns.

- *Listen to your child* (so that your child will listen to you). Particularly as your baby turns into a preschooler and can use words to get your attention, give her some *undivided* attention each day. Practically speaking, you can't offer it every single time she calls for you (nor should you, if you want to foster independence). But make a regular effort to give her your full attention, because as she gets older you'll want her to do the same for you.

Is it true that if my child doesn't learn a foreign language early, it will be much harder later?

If the brain's prime capacity for learning is within the first three years of life, does that mean that as an older child or an adult, your child won't be able to learn certain skills like a foreign language? You have probably seen promotions for foreign language programs aimed at early learners in their "prime"—classes for babies as young as six months are standard. Brain research shows that children do have an easier time learning foreign languages than adults do, particularly in early childhood, as they are learning their native language. But if you can't teach or introduce your child to a foreign language in the first three years of life, the opportunity is not lost forever. Consider that older kids and adults absorb new knowledge all the time. In addition to all the subjects that are introduced in a typical education, not to mention on-the-job learning later in life, we learn many skills from scratch, including foreign languages, playing musical instruments, new computer skills, and much more.

Babies and children may find it easier than their parents or older siblings to learn a foreign language, because their brains are more active in different ways. As the brain matures, the part of the brain that tells languages apart also matures. It's easier for a young brain to take in more than one language without the confusion that arises as our brains develop. But that doesn't mean we can't override that confusion later in life.

Speech and Hearing
How your child communicates

myth

If your child has a speech or language delay, it's nothing to be concerned about, as children usually overcome these problems with age.

reality

Get help early if your child is showing signs of delays in these areas.

the facts

Kids do outgrow some childhood problems, such as certain fears or compulsive behaviors, or physical ailments like some allergies. However, some issues may not vanish with age, and early intervention can make an enormous, positive difference. As a parent, you'll probably be the first adult to notice if your baby or child seems to be having trouble with speech and language. Don't wait until he starts preschool to seek assistance.

Speech and language are not interchangeable terms, particularly when you're talking about delays and problems. "Speech" refers to the quality of sound production, and "language" refers to the content of the communication. However, language doesn't have to consist of recognizable words —if a child produces a nonsense sound in a consistent manner for a specific object or person, then that counts as a "word," even if it is gibberish to others. A child can produce good-quality speech but still have language delays; a different child might have normal language skills but impaired speech, such as stuttering, lisping, or other articulation disorders (like saying "wabbit" for "rabbit"). When a six-month-old doesn't babble or coo, or a two-year-old can't sequence simple words to communicate in a logical way, there could be a language delay or disorder at work. These are some of the most common developmental disabilities among preschool-age children, and early childhood intervention can help. Because language is an indicator of intelligence (and reflects brain development), delayed or abnormal language patterns are considered more serious than speech disorders (such as stuttering, which most children outgrow).

Your pediatrician should ask about your baby or child's overall speech and language development at every regular checkup. These visits become less frequent as your baby grows, however, so you and your caregiver should be observant as your child makes increasing efforts to communicate with speech and language. Here are some general benchmarks to look for. If your baby or child isn't reaching these milestones, talk to your pediatrician.

- *By age three months* Some vocalizing (cooing of vowel sounds should start by three months); recognizes mother's voice (turns head or smiles); may cry differently to communicate different needs

- *By six months* Lots of babbling (consonant sounds); imitates and responds to sounds; repeats certain sounds like "ga," "da," or "ba" (you may hear "mama" or "dada"—sorry, but it's probably unintentional!); laughs; uses speech to communicate different moods (cooing when happy, fussing when displeased)

- *By first birthday* Says "mama" or "dada" in a specific and meaningful way; has a vocabulary of one or more additional words; recognizes his own name; uses pointing to communicate; expresses pleasure or displeasure by using certain sounds or his own "words"; understands the meaning of "no"

- *By second birthday* Speaks in short sentences (two to four words); follows simple directions; tries out lots of new words (often imitated and then mispronounced, which is normal); has more than fifty words and is gaining more and more vocabulary; can point to and name body parts, other people, animals, toys, and everyday objects

- *By third birthday* Can follow directions with two or three steps; uses longer sentences (four to five words or more) and can carry on a conversation; can name most common objects; can make himself understood by strangers

In addition to these benchmarks, apply "the rule of quarters" to speech clarity, as pediatricians do. By age two, children should be 50 percent (or two-quarters) intelligible to strangers; by age three, 75 percent (three-quarters); and by age four, fully intelligible to strangers. The language should be understandable; it need not be perfectly articulated.

Do sippy cups cause lisping?

Some speech pathologists believe that the prolonged use of a sippy cup—a staple in millions of households with thirsty children—can cause lisping, one of the most common speech problems in young children. When a child uses a sippy cup, he positions his tongue toward the roof of his mouth and keeps his lips apart (the same thing happens when he sucks his thumb). In some children, the repetition of this positioning may cause articulation problems such as lisping. Increasingly, speech pathologists are recommending that sippy cup usage be limited to about one month—when going from breast- and/or bottle-feeding to the cup. Instead of cups with spouts, they suggest parents use straws, which require a different positioning of the tongue.

The idea of parting with a sippy cup—the best friend of car upholstery, sofas, and chairs everywhere—after only four weeks may send you groaning as you stock up on paper towels. But increasingly, this theory is gaining in popularity and will probably be the subject of more research. Talk to your pediatrician about the latest recommendations, especially if your child uses such a cup. (And my crystal ball tells me that before long, sippy-cup makers will offer parents "speech-friendly" versions of their products!)

myth

You should correct your toddler's mispronunciations.

reality

At this stage, modeling clear speech—without correcting your toddler's—is all you need to do.

the facts

Many toddlers love to "talk"—to themselves, to one another, to grown-ups, and to anyone who will listen. They are often imitating adult speech patterns, trying out new sounds and inflections, and attempting to get their tongues around countless words they are hearing for the first time. Many parents still recall the toddler lexicon in their own household. One of our daughters loved "totton tandy" (cotton candy)—she had trouble with her hard *c* pronunciation, which is not uncommon. Kids will drop letters or syllables ("school" is "cool"), add things where they don't belong, double up on words ("milk" is "milky-milk"), or do other normal things as they strive to master more words and build their budding vocabularies. So, should you correct your toddler each time she says "sue" for "shoe"?

If your child is developing normally and using language logically (see the guidelines on pages 187–188), it's okay to let the mispronunciations go for now. Constant correction may actually frustrate her and make her struggle even more, or discourage her from trying out new words. (Think how you would feel if you were trying to learn a new skill and someone was constantly correcting your every effort.) Speak clearly to her (reading and singing are great opportunities for her to absorb and try out new words in a fun environment), but don't expect her to be able to do the same, particularly if she hasn't yet reached her third birthday.

If you use "baby talk" you may be hindering her speech at this point, so model correct pronunciation to assist her, and do so in a benign and helpful way, not in a disapproving, corrective manner. Simply repeat her mispronunciation the correct way. When she says, "Daddy, can I have totten tandy?" you can respond with, "You want cotton candy? Sure." (I know it isn't the healthiest treat, but if you're at the circus . . .)

Clear pronunciation takes longer for some children— often till age three or four; even among some kindergarteners, mispronunciations linger. If your child's hearing is okay and she understands how to use language, and how to respond to the language you use with her, chances are her mispronunciations are nothing to worry about. The parts of the mouth that control speech (the tongue, the lips, the palate) are still developing and growing stronger. Right now, her mind is working faster and more efficiently than her mouth—but the speech production parts of her mouth will eventually catch up.

If you are concerned that the problem goes beyond typical toddler mispronunciation—if she's truly showing signs of a language delay or if it's a more significant speech problem — talk to your pediatrician about further evaluation and possible speech therapy. I often ask concerned parents if they can think of another adult with the same speech problem their child has. If the answer is no, the speech problem will likely be resolved, either on its own or with some intervention.

myth
The youngest child in a large family will be a late talker.

reality
Birth order can play a role in speech and language, but is not always a deciding factor.

the facts
It makes sense on the surface. A child bringing up the rear in a family of more than two siblings talks less—because he doesn't have to. He has at least two "helpers" (in addition to parents and caregivers) who understand him and intuit what he wants, even if he doesn't speak, or doesn't speak clearly. These helpers are always present, playing with him, eating when he eats, and running interference between him and the grown-up in charge. They've been around Mom and Dad—especially the oldest one—longer than him, so they've had more exposure to adult language. Furthermore, there's so much racket all the time that he can't get a "bye-bye" or "me want" in edgewise. Right? Well, not always.

There is some evidence that factors such as birth order, gender, and genetics do play a role in speech and language development, but because no two children develop the exact same way, it's best to think of these things as *possible* factors and not *determining* factors. A toddler girl may speak before her same-age male playmate—or he may be the chatterbox in their play group. The youngest child in a family of several siblings may talk a little later than his big brothers or sisters, but he may also talk early—because he is constantly "communicating" with other children who like to teach him new words. It depends on the household itself, the personalities of the siblings, the amount and quality of time a child spends with other children and adults, and much more.

Don't assume that a child is destined to develop a certain way based on a single factor like birth order. The problem with assuming that "last child equals late talker" is that if that youngest sibling truly is having a language delay, he won't get the early intervention that could make the difference. Clinically significant language delays are not due to birth order.

myth

You can't effectively test a baby's hearing until after one year of age.

reality

A hearing test can and should be performed on a baby in the first month of life.

the facts

A baby's hearing can be tested soon after birth. In fact, the AAP recommends that all newborns receive a hearing screening before they come home from the hospital (these painless procedures can be done in minutes, while an infant is sleeping). About two to three out of every thousand children in the United States are born deaf or with some hearing loss. The cause could be genetic, or an in utero infection such as herpes, toxoplasmosis, or rubella; in some cases, there is no explanation. Babies with a congenital hearing loss who receive early intervention (before six months) can eventually develop language skills equal to those of other children. If a baby fails a hearing test, an audiologist will perform further evaluations to determine the extent of the loss and to help devise treatment options. Newborns who are not screened at birth should receive a screening within the first three months of life.

A baby may be born with normal hearing, but could have some hearing loss later during childhood. Some causes include head injuries, persistent ear infections with effusion (fluid that will not drain), infections such as chicken pox or meningitis, or exposure to damaging noise levels. If your child is not hitting standard benchmarks for language development (see pages 187–188), her hearing should be checked. Sometimes, an observant day care provider or preschool teacher may notice a pattern that indicates a hearing problem, but it's likely that you'll notice it first. Note that unilateral hearing loss (occurring in one ear only) is difficult to detect without testing because a child will still respond well to sound; he can still hear normally with one ear.

As with language delays, the key is early intervention. Check with your pediatrician to find out if and how she screens babies and children for normal hearing. Some day care providers, preschools, and school systems offer free or low-cost hearing screenings.

Vision
Bringing the facts into focus

myth
Children usually outgrow "crossed eyes" (strabismus).

reality
Left untreated, this condition can persist and lead to serious vision problems.

the facts

A baby is born with peripheral vision, but it takes some time for her to learn to focus on a single object in front of her, and her ability to distinguish between colors can take about four months. This is why many toys for newborns feature strong black-and-white patterns, or high-contrast colors, designed for very young eyes.

In the first weeks and months of life, her still-maturing eyes may "wander" and she may appear to look cross-eyed or wall-eyed (one or both eyes drift outward, as opposed to inward for cross-eyes). This is because the eye muscles are still strengthening and learning to work together. If you notice that this wandering condition does not resolve by age four months, inform your pediatrician. Your baby may have "strabismus," an inability to focus on a single point because the eyes are not working together, resulting in cross-eye, or wall eye. There are six muscles that connect to each eye; some may be weaker or stronger in one eye, and this muscle imbalance causes the strabismus, or wandering. (Strabismus may also have a genetic component, or it can be related to other medical conditions, such as Down syndrome.)

Don't wait for this condition to correct on its own if it persists beyond four months, since it can lead to "lazy eye," where the stronger eye begins to dominate as the affected eye grows even weaker. In some cases, partial loss of vision or even blindness in the weak eye can result. Treatment begins with an evaluation by a pediatric ophthalmologist and can involve special eye drops, eye patches, eye glasses, eye exercises, and, in some cases, corrective surgery to adjust muscle tension or address other problems, like a cataract. If your older baby or child suddenly develops strabismus, see your doctor right away.

Your baby's eyes should be examined at birth (as with hearing screenings, the AAP recommends that this take place in the hospital before you bring your newborn home) and during routine well-baby visits up to age six months. At age three, your child should have another vision screening, and another one at around age five or when she starts kindergarten. Your pediatrician will do informal screenings during routine physicals; he may be equipped to do more thorough eye exams or may refer you to a pediatric ophthalmologist. Even if your child shows no sign of vision problems, it's important to have regular preventive screenings.

Is it true that eyes can get "stuck" if you cross them on purpose?

"Don't cross your eyes! They'll stay that way!" It may have worked on you as a kid, but you can't truthfully use this one on your child, since it's an old wives' tale. When your child (or you, if you're feeling dextrous) crosses her eyes on purpose, she's moving muscles that control her eye movement. These muscles won't "lock" or otherwise get stuck (in fact, it takes effort to keep them in that position); as with any muscles, she may tire them out a bit, but she is not doing any permanent damage to her eyes while she holds them in this comical or unsettling, but temporary, position. (Of course, even though it's not *true*, it might do the trick if you want to discourage her from looking like Jerry Lewis!)

myth

Don't let your child sit too close to the television or he'll damage his eyes.

reality

Sitting close to the TV won't hurt your child's vision.

the facts

There are many reasons to move your child away from the television set (see the box on pages 197–198), but the reason your mother gave you ("Don't sit so close or you'll hurt your eyes!") isn't one of them.

Your child's young eyes can handle up-close focusing without the strain you might feel, and his neck can probably handle the strain better, too. (The first row at your local movie theater is usually a grown-up-free zone.) Older generations who ushered in the living room television set were probably suspicious about this electrical device that emitted so much power. "Don't sit so close to the TV" was probably first uttered in the 1950s. However, there is no scientific or medical evidence to suggest a television screen emits any vision-damaging lights or electrical rays.

Older eyes grow tired from focusing for too long (the same thing happens when we sit and stare at the computer screen—and it's no surprise that kids can do it longer without feeling the strain), but there is no risk to vision skills.

If your child is nearsighted, he may simply see the picture better when he sits closer to the set. Nearsightedness (myopia) usually occurs later in life, but some children may develop myopia in the second or third year of life. If your child consistently sits close to the TV so that he can see the picture better, if he holds books close to his face, if he squints or shows other signs of having difficulty focusing on objects in the distance, he may need corrective lenses. Because the eyes change as they grow, the prescription should be checked every six months. (And make sure your child isn't sitting up close because he has a hearing problem—not a vision problem!)

How much TV should a child watch?

The AAP recommends that children under two not watch television at all—including DVDs or videos. How realistic is this for some families, particularly when the TV is centrally located in a house and older siblings (and parents) like to watch? The reality is that nearly 75 percent of all children under the age of two have watched some television, according to research from the Kaiser Family Foundation. Between the ages of two and six, more than 75 percent of children are turning the TV on by themselves.

The arguments against television (as well as DVD/videos) are well known. If a child is exposed to advertising messages, violence, substance abuse, sexuality, and other adult content, studies have shown that there will be negative effects on behavior. Television viewing has also been linked to childhood obesity. Most studies have not focused on children under age two. Nevertheless, the AAP reminds us that the early years are a crucial time for parent-child bonding as well as intellectual and physical development, and time spent in front of a television set can interfere with these important goals.

Like many parents, you will search for ways to balance reality with such recommendations, particularly as your child can figure out the remote and find the power button. Start with these tips:

Set limits. The AAP suggests no more than one to two hours per day maximum (including videos/DVDs) for children two and older.

Watch with your child. You should always know what your child is watching. Sharing the experience will also allow you to have discussions about favorite stories and characters, lessons learned, and more.

Don't put a television set in your child's room. If you allow a TV in his room when he's very young, and try to take it away later so that he can concentrate on homework or go to sleep on time (or so you can monitor what and how much he's watching), you'll have a battle on your hands. Interestingly, and if you need more convincing, researchers have noted lower standardized test scores in math, reading, and language arts among third-graders who had televisions in their bedrooms.

Look for quality content. Search for educational content and wholesome stories when you choose programming and DVDs/videos. As with books, move up to more stimulating and interesting content as your child matures.

Finally, consider the example you may be setting with regard to TV watching. (And don't forget all that time you may log on your home computer, which your child may be noticing more and more—to a very young child, it may appear to be just another form of TV.) Make sure your own actions are consistent with the message you want to send to your child.

myth

Holding books too close to your child's eyes will damage her vision.

reality

It won't damage her vision, although it may indicate near-sightedness.

the facts

As with sitting close to the television or computer screen, there is no evidence that holding books or other reading material close to the eyes will damage the vision, although it may tire the eye muscles. If your child can look at books or pictures only this way, however, have her checked for nearsightedness. (See pages 196–197.)

You can't cause nearsightedness by looking at objects up close, because it's usually the result of how the eyeball is shaped. With normal vision, the eyeballs are spherical; with nearsighted or myopic vision, the eyeball is elongated. Similarly, farsightedness (or hyperopia), which makes it difficult to see objects when they are up close, is also usually due to how the eyeball is shaped—in this case, it's somewhat shorter than normal. Many children are born farsighted, but as they grow and the eyeball grows too, this condition goes away. Unlike myopia, farsighted vision rarely needs to be corrected with lenses unless the condition is severe.

myth

If your child plays or looks at books in insufficient light, he'll hurt his eyes.

reality

Reading, working, or playing in low light will not hurt vision.

the facts

Once again, as with watching television, staring at a computer screen, squinting, or crossing the eyes, your child's eyes may get tired, but she won't damage them by looking at a book in low light or sitting in a dim room watching television.

Low light doesn't damage vision, "wear out" the eyes, or cause nearsightedness. (See pages 74–75 for information regarding the effects of night-lights on vision.) Your child may simply not realize that turning on more lights will make it easier to see his book or work on the picture he's drawing. (If he seems sensitive to normal light, talk to your pediatrician.) As he gets older and attempts reading under the covers with a flashlight, you can discourage him for other reasons—such as sleep deprivation—but there's no truth in saying, "Don't read in the dark or you'll hurt your eyes!"

Walking
from first steps to first shoes

myth
A mobile infant walker will help your child walk faster.

reality
Mobile walkers do more harm than good.

the facts
Mobile walkers, wheeled devices designed to help babies zoom from point A to point B before they can do so on their own two feet, are dangerous—so dangerous that the American Academy of Pediatrics called for a total ban on their manufacturing in 2001 and again in 2006, because of the injuries and even fatalities they have caused over the years. Babies can push themselves to the edges of stairways and fall down, resulting in head injuries, as well as

broken bones and bruises. Babies can also get into trouble exploring—going into kitchens, bathrooms, or other areas of a home and encountering such hazards as hot stoves, toilets, sharp corners, hard surfaces, and other dangers like drawers or cabinets containing items that could injure them. Walkers have been known to tip over when they hit the edge of a rug or a bump in the floor surface.

Parents continue to buy walkers, many of which have been redesigned to meet new safety standards. There are many reasons for this, including the belief that babies who use walkers will learn to walk sooner. In fact, just the opposite is true. Research has shown that babies in walkers may become overly dependent on the devices and be reluctant to walk unassisted. In one study cited by the AAP, babies between the ages of six and eighteen months sat, crawled, and walked *later* than babies who did not spend time in walkers. Furthermore, walkers strengthen the wrong muscle groups for walking and balancing—the lower leg muscles as opposed to the hips and upper legs.

Some manufacturers of walkers have taken steps to make these devices safer, by adding braking systems that are triggered if one wheel goes over a step, and by widening walkers so that they don't go through standard thirty-six-inch doorways. Because there is no evidence that walkers help babies get ready for walking, and because the dangers outweigh any benefit (despite the newer safety features, which not all manufacturers offer), the AAP still recommends against their use.

So, what's a good alternative for a baby who wants to be upright but can't walk, and parents who would like a safe "station" for their increasingly active baby? Many parents like such devices as "Exersaucers" (the actual brand name for one such "activity center" made by Evenflo), which are like walkers without wheels. A baby can stand, bounce, and swivel around as she plays with objects in a plastic tray that encircles the activity center. These stationary activity centers are safe because the baby can't go anywhere and is limited to the toys that are within her reach.

However, that doesn't mean she shouldn't have adult supervision, which is vital at *all* times, whether you choose an Exersaucer-type device, a bouncy seat, a swing, or other type of activity center. Make sure that your baby is old enough to use any such gear you bring into your home. For instance, babies should be able to sit up on their own to use stationary activity centers, but newborns can go into cradle-type swings and most bouncy seats. Don't let your baby sit in a stationary activity center for extended periods of time, as she should be allowed and encouraged to scoot, crawl, cruise, and stand on her own. These are all steps that lead to unassisted walking (though some babies may scoot less, cruise more, or not crawl at all—such variations are normal, too—see the box on pages 204–205, for more on stages that lead to walking).

myth

Buy the best shoes that you can afford for your toddler, such as leather high-tops with good ankle support.

reality

Choose wisely, but you don't need to spend a lot of money to find appropriate footwear for your new walker.

the facts

Once upon a time, there were children's shoe stores like the local Stride-Rite on Main Street (which still exists, though it has moved to the mall), where baby got his first pair of Buster Browns—often white leather, hard-soled high-tops, the classic baby shoe that was often bronzed for the grandparents.

Given how inflexible and rigid those old-fashioned shoes were, they were probably better off bronzed than on baby's feet. Now baby shoes have gone high-end. Parents can spend astounding sums of money on a pair of size four toddler shoes made in Italy, with breathable leather uppers, lots of arch and ankle support, and padded insoles. But do newly walking baby feet do better in designer or high-tech footwear?

We now know that in cultures where children are allowed to go barefoot, their feet develop more strength and flexibility. When children go barefoot, which they should be allowed to do, they learn to grip with their toes and build important muscles in the arch. Contrary to what many shoe manufacturers would have you think, fancy footwear with built-in arch support is not necessary for a new walker. An older child or an adult may need arch support, but not a new walker. Babies and very young children have plump feet, but they do have arches—this curve, however, is not apparent because of the fat in the arch area. Ankle support, which those old-fashioned high-tops provided and which newer high-backed styles offer, is also not necessary for a new walker, and is probably downright uncomfortable. Little feet grow strong and healthy when they are left in their natural state—bare.

Of course, going barefoot is not practical when the temperature drops or if there are hazards on the floor that could injure a new walker's soft feet; going barefoot outside is also a tricky proposition, unless you're on a pristine beach or lawn. If you're indoors and it's chilly, slipper socks or cloth booties with nonskid soles are a good bet. If you want something more substantial than slipper-type footwear, any softly constructed shoes with nonskid soles, such as inexpensive canvas sneakers, are fine. Because you'll probably replace shoes every few months, there's no point in investing a lot of money in shoes for the new walker. Many parents like to buy one half-size up. As long as the shoe isn't so big that it causes slippage or stumbling, this is a good tip—there's no question that your child is going to grow into that next half size. (For more information on infants and footwear, see pages 91–92.)

Always have your child's foot measured, particularly if you haven't bought shoes in a few months. (You'll want to do this throughout their childhood—feet seem to have their own growth spurts!) As your baby grows out of the new walker phase and there are more shoe options available, you still don't have to spend a lot on shoes. All things being equal, go for the best value, not the brand. A good fit, safety, and comfort should be at the top of your list. Soon enough, style may be your child's priority, so save your pennies for when they just have to have the pink flowery boots or the basketball shoes that light up.

When will my baby walk?

A baby usually takes her first steps around her first birthday, but there are always early walkers and late walkers. As long as she's hitting the following milestones, all systems are go. If she is not progressing along these lines, talk to your pediatrician.

Getting into a sitting position   Babies sit up on their own between four and seven months—and then they topple over. Between eight and twelve months, they learn to get themselves into a sitting position on their own and stay there.

Crawling (or scooting and slithering)   Off they go. Now that they're able to get on all fours, they figure out forward motion (and sometimes backward motion, too). Babies crawl between seven and ten months. Some babies love crawling, and others do it briefly and then move on to more upright challenges. And some babies don't crawl at all—they scoot around on their bottoms, they slither on their bellies, and they find other ways to get moving. However she does it, the main goal is for your baby to coordinate arm and leg motion on both sides of her body, which she'll need to be able to do for walking.

Pulling into a standing position Up she goes—usually by grabbing on to you or a handy piece of furniture. Make sure furniture is secure and heavy enough for your baby to pull on—now is when the importance of baby-proofing really comes into play!.

"Cruising" She "walks" by holding on to furniture. Her stroll may consist of the length of the living room sofa, but she's getting ready.

Stands without support Look, Ma, no hands! She'll stand without holding on to anything for a few moments at a time. Very exciting for her, and for you.

First steps The big moment is here! She'll go from unassisted standing to a few forward steps. Now there's no going back—before you know it, she'll want to see the world. Hide the car keys!

myth

Shoes can help your baby walk sooner.

reality

Wearing shoes won't expedite the walking process.

the facts

Remember those high-top shoes I mentioned in the previous myth? One reason they were once so popular is that previous generations of parents (and yes, probably some pediatricians) believed that putting a toddler in shoes would help children walk at an earlier age. Of course, we know now that that is far from true and that children hit several developmental milestones before they walk (see the box on pages 204–205, "When will my baby walk?"). Shoes have nothing to do with when they hit these milestones, and in fact, babies need to be able to grip with their toes, flex their feet, and strengthen their muscles before they can walk—tasks that are more easily accomplished when the feet are bare.

Should you put your child into shoes as soon as she is walking? Not necessarily. Barefoot (or in skid-proof booties or socks) is still best if she's indoors at home and walking on a safe surface. Shoes are meant for when she's outside and in the elements, or walking on an indoor surface where she'll need protection (like a less-than-pristine basement floor) or in a public place like a store.

Many parents worry when their toddlers insist on wearing the same pair of shoes over and over again. "Isn't it bad for her feet if she wears her sneakers/sandals/cowboy boots/dress-up shoes every single day?" Toddlers develop rigid desires and dislikes when it comes to things like shoes. Unless the shoes are inappropriate for the weather or the surface that she's walking on, are too big, or no longer fit, it's unlikely that wearing the same pair of shoes will cause conditions like flat feet or bunions, in part because a new walker's feet grow so quickly that she's on to a new pair of shoes before such conditions can develop (and even if she insists on the same style, you can relax if the shoe is comfortable and safe and has the proper fit). Make sure to have your child's feet measured each time you buy new shoes.

Physical Growth
Big, little, and in between

myth
A baby's length at birth is predictive of adult height.

reality

Length at birth is not a predictor, but later measurements may be.

the facts

There's no question that genes play a role in what heights we may ultimately reach as adults, but at birth, it's too soon to tell. A baby with very tall parents may be unusually "long" at birth—or not. However, one of the more accurate predictors is a toddler's height at age two. We know that most people achieve half their adult height at age two, so you can multiply your child's height at his second birthday by two, and roughly estimate his adult height. Then again, not every single person fits into this pattern, since illness or other factors can have an impact on growth. And truly, the age-two formula is give or take a few inches; it's not precise (nor are other predictive measurements, like foot size).

In recent years, many parenting Web sites have added "estimate your child's adult height" calculators, where parents can plug in their child's age, height, and weight, and their own heights, to obtain a rough measure of adult height. You'll notice, however, that these tools come with such disclaimers as "this is just a best-guess estimate," since it's virtually impossible to know, without a doubt, how tall or short your child may be. If you want to do this calculation yourself, here's the "mid-parental height formula" used by pediatricians: Determine the average of the two parents' heights (mother plus father, divided by two) and then add 2.5 inches for boys and subtract 2.5 inches for girls. Make sure Dad gives his real height—in one study, parents (especially fathers) overestimated their heights!

These predictions can be fun to play with—or they can be unsettling if you're concerned about your child's growth.

If you have any questions about your child's growth—whether it seems rapid or slow—don't do the math yourself; talk to your pediatrician.

myth

"Growing pains" are caused by the growth of bones and joints.

reality

Growing pains are real, but in young children they are muscular aches, not bone- or joint-related.

the facts

Your preschooler, who is having a bit of a growth spurt, may wake up at night telling you that her legs hurt. There is no redness or swelling, she can walk normally, and she has no pain in other limbs, joints, or parts of her body. There's a good chance she's having typical (benign) growing pains. These are actually muscle aches.

For immediate relief, gentle massage, stretching, and a heating pad (used safely) can ease the aches, which don't last long and usually don't hit during the day.

Benign growing pains usually occur between three and five years of age and then return between eight and ten years of age. If your child is experiencing persistent leg or other limb pain during the day, is having trouble with walking or other normal movements, has joint pain, stiffness, swelling, or redness, or any other symptoms that don't seem related to benign growing pain, see your pediatrician to rule out such conditions as Lyme disease, a viral or bacterial infection, or juvenile rheumatoid arthritis, which occurs between the ages of three and six when growing pains are also common.

myth

Some children are double-jointed.

reality

No child (or adult) is "double-jointed," but kids can do some eye-popping things with their growing bodies.

the facts

Remember that kid in grade school who could bend her thumb to her wrist? Or that college friend who could loop his leg around his neck? That's where you probably first heard the term "double-jointed," and now your child is doing some pretty amazing things with his left index finger. But he's not double-jointed, which suggests that there are two joints, and not just one. He may, however, have "hypermobility," meaning that he has unusual flexibility. Hypermobility most often occurs in joints located in the fingers, legs, or arms. This condition is benign, although it can be associated with some medical conditions or developmental delays. If you're concerned, talk to your pediatrician.

Particularly as they grow older, children enjoy showing off all the cool things their bodies can do—even if some of these feats involve socially unacceptable sights and sounds (burping on command, the ever popular flatulence sound produced by the hand in the armpit). Usually they won't do any lasting damage (cracking the knuckles does not cause arthritis). As mentioned above, if you're concerned about any of the extraordinary feats your child may be able to do with his body, talk to his doctor—but usually things like finger-popping or ear-wiggling turn out to be a source of amusement (until they become a source of annoyance), and not a cause for concern.

Behavior
The good, the bad, and the normal

myth
Time-outs don't work.

reality
When done consistently, a time-out can be an effective way to manage unacceptable behavior.

the facts
If a child is repeatedly doing something unacceptable—not just annoying, but dangerous and destructive, like being cruel to a pet, climbing on an unstable piece of furniture, or fighting beyond the norm with a playmate or sibling—you can use time-outs (removing the child from the situation for a specific amount of time as a penalty, and to allow him to regroup) to help curb the behavior you don't want. But you have to be consistent and follow some basic steps. You'll need a quiet, safe area for the time-out spot and a kitchen timer.

■ Make sure your child knows that what she is doing is unacceptable. Time-outs aren't meant for single episodes of unacceptable behavior; they are effective if a child repeatedly engages in an action you want to bring to a halt. Don't swoop down without a verbal warning (unless she is causing or entering into a dangerous situation). Give one clear warning and be explicit that the consequence will be a time-out. (For example, "Don't pull your sister's hair again or you will get a time-out.") If she doesn't stop, state that she is going into a time-out because she did not do what was requested. Don't engage in further conversation.

■ In advance, you should have designated an appropriate and safe place to send her for the time-out. A toy-filled room where she can happily entertain herself is not a good choice. A quiet, boring spot in the dining room is.

■ Once your child has removed herself (or you have physically removed her, with care) from the scene of the bad behavior to the designated time-out spot, start the timer. Experts recommend one minute of time for each year of the child's age, but less time can be effective with some kids.

■ Do not argue, explain, or negotiate. You have already warned your child that her behavior would result in a time-out; you have stated that she is now going to have a time-out because she didn't change the behavior. Leave it at that. Start the timer and disengage from your child (some parents find that they benefit from the time-out, too, as it gives them a chance to calm down). You may leave an older child alone, but use common sense. A very young child needs supervision. You can do a time-out with children as young as one year of age, and you may even need to hold a small toddler on your lap. But don't interact normally or there's no point in the time-out.

■ Once your child has calmed down and the time on the clock is up, steer her toward a new activity. Don't dwell on her unacceptable behavior and don't lecture. By moving on, you're sending a signal that you trust your child to do better next time. If your child is old enough, have a constructive conversation about what she did wrong later on, when you've both gotten some distance from the incident.

Time-outs are remarkably effective with most children, but they may have little to no impact on some, particularly if they are done inconsistently.

When it comes to discipline, there is no one-size-fits-all approach. You know your child better than anyone, so if time-outs don't work in your household, you should look at other styles of discipline that suit her (and your own) personality. Withholding privileges and using consequences are other alternatives; the main point is to pick an age-appropriate

response that fits the bad behavior. Don't overdo the consequence, or underplay the bad behavior.

The three biggest parenting pitfalls when it comes to discipline are not being predictable, not being immediate, and
not being consistent. *Predictable* means that the child has
been warned of the consequence; *immediate* means that the
problem is dealt with at the time that it's observed, not days
or hours later; and *consistent* means that it happens each
and every time it is supposed to happen. Parents sometimes
balk at giving their kids a time-out in public—it's a hassle to
leave the supermarket when your cart is full, or you're in the
middle of a playdate at a friend's house. If the child is doing
something unacceptable, by not invoking the time-out, the
adult forgoes being predictable and immediate. If the adult
tries to use a time-out the next day, when the same behavior
flares up, the adult is being inconsistent. When the adult is
consistent, however, behavior management can be extremely
effective.

If you need more help

If you are having trouble coming up with an effective way
to manage your child's undesirable behavior, you don't
have to go it alone—particularly if you feel that the situation is getting increasingly difficult or serious. Talk to your
pediatrician, who may provide you with helpful suggestions
or refer you to a behavioral psychologist or other expert.

I like to tell parents that sometimes, as with exercise,
some people benefit from a personal trainer to help them
meet their goals while ensuring that their efforts are reason-
able, appropriate, and healthy; others can reach their goals
on their own, especially through educating themselves on
the topic.

Often, with some perspective and guidance, you can land upon strategies that work just through reading some of the better books out there on behavior management. Following are some of the titles that many parents (myself included) have found helpful over the years.

1-2-3 Magic: Effective Discipline for Children 2–12 by Thomas W. Phelan, Ph.D., 2003 (Parentmagic Inc.).

S.O.S.: Help for Parents, 3rd edition by Lynn Clark and John Robb, 2005 (Parents Press).

Parenting the Strong-Willed Child: The Clinically Proven Five-Week Program for Parents of Two- to Six-Year-Olds by Rex Forehand, Ph.D., and Nicholas Long, Ph.D., 2002 (McGraw-Hill).

Your Defiant Child: Eight Steps to Better Behavior by Russell A. Barkley, Ph.D., and Christine M. Benton, 1998 (Guilford).

myth

It's never too early to teach the importance of sharing.

reality

Children need to be mature enough to understand concepts like sharing, which doesn't come naturally to toddlers.

the facts

Have you ever watched toddlers playing "together"? They don't really have a lot of social and physical interaction, but they do engage in something called "parallel play," meaning that they simply play separately, but side-by-side. Things can continue fairly peacefully until one child decides he wants what the other child has—and then the age-old toddler battle cry rings out across the playground: *"MINE!"*

Babies, toddlers, and preschoolers are very possessive of everything, from their toys to their parents. But at a certain point it is important to introduce the concept of sharing. Generally you can start to do this at around age two. If you try it sooner, you'll just wind up with a lot of tearful toddlers, as they aren't really developmentally ready for this concept. Consider what an enormous idea it is for a toddler to accept—someone is going to take something precious from him (or ask him to hand it over), and how does he know that he'll ever see that stuffed animal, wooden spoon, or balloon ever again? This is major!

Start by setting a good example. Share your own "toys"— let him hold your cell phone or wristwatch, but make it clear that you're "sharing" and not giving it to him forever. Ask him if you can borrow a marker or look at one of his books. Try simple games where you can take turns—whether you're alternating stacking blocks to make a tower, or having a tea party and sharing pretend cookies (or real ones). Show him that sharing can double his fun.

Let him get some practice with someone his own size. By age two, your child may start to make "friends"— maybe in the neighborhood or at day care. Even if he has siblings (and unless he is a twin), he needs some experience learning to share with children his own age. Host a playdate so that he can share on his own turf, take him to play at a friend's house so he can be "the guest," or let him bring a toy to share with new friends at a playground.

Reward his efforts. "Thank you!" goes a long way. Your child wants to please you, and if you respond to his sharing efforts—however minor they may be at first—with a positive reaction, you'll reinforce his good behavior. If he's playing with a friend, admire their sharing skills.

Don't expect too much too soon. Sharing is a learned behavior and it can take years before some kids get it down. Even then, there may be some prized items that your child will never share, and that's normal, too. (Even we adults have a few "hands-off" possessions.) Never take something precious away from your child—like a favorite doll or blanket—and give it to another child just to make your point. Your child will be hurt and confused. If he has something special that he does not want a playmate to handle, help him put the item safely away before his friend arrives.

In the years to come, preschool and kindergarten teachers will emphasize sharing skills, but for now, starting at around age two, you can plant the seeds at home. Just don't expect a whole tree to grow in a short time.

Does spanking work?

Spanking was once a widespread practice and an accepted form of discipline, but times have changed. We know now that spanking may work in the short term, but it doesn't stop the bad behavior for good or have any long-term benefits. It also is a physically aggressive and hurtful act, it can lead to escalating physical struggles if a child chooses to fight back or flee, and it can cause children to become angry or fearful of their parents, whom they may come to view as bullies. It also teaches children that it's acceptable to humiliate or cause pain in others (try teaching a child who is spanked that he should not hit other children). Adults who were spanked as children have been shown to be violent and more physically aggressive than their peers. For all these reasons, the AAP recommends that spanking not be used as a method of discipline; most but not all pediatricians agree with the AAP on this policy statement.

myth

Children of working mothers/stay-at-home mothers are happier and do better overall.

reality

How a child turns out does not hinge on whether a parent works or stays home.

the facts

It's hard to dodge the "mommy wars" these days—even though more than half of all U.S. mothers work outside the home, either full-time or part-time. Choosing to work or to stay with a child is a very personal decision, and there is no one-size-fits-all answer. There is also no reason to pass judgment on one view or the other; ultimately, it's the *quality of the parenting*—not who is spending more hours with a child during the day—that determines the well-being of a child.

Though dads work too, the "to work or not to work" argument traditionally swirls around moms, who are more likely than fathers to give up their work after the birth of a child. If a mother wants to work (out of necessity or desire), she won't be happy at home all day. If a mother chooses to stay home with a child and is satisfied with that decision, she won't be happy if she goes to a job that separates her from her child. Children do best when parents are satisfied with the decisions they make about work, and when they are cared for by an engaged and loving adult, whether that person is a parent or another caregiver.

A few years ago, some initial results of a major, ongoing study being conducted by the National Institute of Child Health and Human Development were released to the public. One piece of news dominated all others: some portions of the study indicated that children who spent more than thirty hours a week in center-based child care were more "aggressive" than children who were cared for at home (or in smaller settings).

However, the study—the largest study every undertaken on the impact of early child care, and which has been tracking over 1,300 children from birth since 1991—also pointed out that this behavior was noted only by teachers and not by other adults; furthermore, the aggressive characteristics declined and all but disappeared as children progressed from early childhood into grade school. The study also showed that children in quality child care had more "school readiness" skills (in areas of literacy and math) than children who were cared for at home, and were more independent in many areas.

You may have a close relative such as a parent, in-law, or grandparent from another generation (or even a friend from your own generation) who repeatedly shares the opinion that a child is always better off being taken care of by Mom (or Dad) than by another caregiver. That is a myth. Your child is better off in a quality situation that works for you and your family.

To get a free booklet for parents based on the NICHD study, visit http://www.nichd.nih.gov/publications and locate "The NICHD Study of Early Child Care and Youth Development (SECCYD): Findings for Children up to Age 4½ Years." You'll find interesting information on how children are affected by working or at-home parents, as well as information on what constitutes quality child care.

myth
Girls are shy; boys are rambunctious.

reality

Gender is not the only determining factor when it comes to behavior and personality.

the facts

"Oh, he's such a boy!" "She's such a girly-girl!"

We know that gender affects how children develop and behave. For instance, girls often talk sooner than boys and are more social at an early age; boys are sometimes more physical than girls and may have better spatial relationship skills. However, despite such differences between the sexes, toddlers, preschoolers, and young children don't always fall into neat categories of his or her behavior. There are plenty of quiet, wallflower boys out there, just as there are lots of physically strong and "wild" girls—and there is nothing developmentally wrong with young children who don't behave along traditionally drawn gender lines.

Adults—often without meaning to—tend to steer very young children into their gender roles, though it's not really until about age three, when increased socialization with peers begins and nature kicks in, that kids start to make their own gender-specific choices. Up till that point, boys are often happy to play with dolls and dress in a big sister's princess costume, and girls think nothing of crashing toy trucks together or trying to jump off the top of the slide. As the third birthday approaches, however, increasingly "girls will be girls" and "boys will be boys."

A preschooler may observe Mom cooking a meal or Dad carrying a hammer. These observations are filed away and may emerge later when this child plays house—a girl may want to imitate her mother, and a boy his father. Other adults add to this reinforcement of traditional roles. A boy will receive trucks and trains for his birthday, while a girl gets dolls and a tea set. Children begin to have more same-sex playmates at this age (by choice, or maybe just because parents of same-age sons or daughters become friendly and start a play group). Though the two sexes may still play together, boys will start to engage in more physical games and perhaps get a baseball glove as a present, and girls will start to mature socially and may be drawn to more feminine toys, particularly if they are presented as the main choices. Adults smile and approve of the little girl pushing her doll in the stroller, and of the little boy who pretends to be a superhero fighting the bad guys. And peers may start to make fun of the gentle boy who still wants to take care of "sick" stuffed animals, and of the "tomboy" girl who hates pink and loves to run fast.

By the time kids start school, they have a good sense of how they are supposed to behave as girls or as boys, even if their parents have not drawn such rigid lines between the genders. Most will find pleasure in being who they are as their gender identities take hold. If your child is three or four and strongly resists and rejects normal gender behavior (a boy who still wants to dress as a girl; a girl who is distressed and sad that she was born female), talk to your pediatrician.

Yes, some girls *are* shy and some boys *are* rambunctious, but sometimes little girls will be boys, little boys will be girls, and that's okay.

myth
An only child is lonely and self-centered.

reality
An only child can grow into a well-adjusted and happy adult, as can any child.

the facts
"Oh, she's an only child—that's why she acts so spoiled/ bossy/dependent."

There are many myths and stereotypes about only children: They are self-centered because they don't have to share their parents (or their toys) with siblings. They are lonely or quiet because they spend so much time by themselves. They are high-achieving prodigies because their parents focus so much attention on them. They are not competitive. They are "people-pleasers."

Only children, however, don't grow up in a vacuum. They develop and grow like other children. They have peer groups and friends their own age. They aren't isolated from the rest of society.

In fact, studies have shown that only children from two-parent families often have a slight edge on children with siblings. Many "singletons" score higher on standardized tests, are better educated, and go on to achieve more professional success than other children. (Some famous onlies include Elvis, former Federal Reserve chairman Alan Greenspan, Elizabeth Taylor, Tiger Woods, Winston Churchill, playwright Lillian Hellman, and Leonardo da Vinci.)

Parents are likely to have more time (and money) to spend on their only children—but many still worry that their kids are missing out by not having a brother or a sister (or both). If you're the parent of an only child and you've made the choice to stop at one (by design or by necessity), there are many simple steps you can take to allay your concerns. Here are some things to consider.

■ *Make sure your child gets enough time with children her own age.* Children learn some of their most important lessons from other children. Eventually, your child will start school and be around other kids all day, every day. But before that happens, make sure she's getting adequate time in play groups, at preschool, on the playground, and with other kids like her.

■ *Resist the temptation of giving all the time.* Just because you can doesn't mean you should—and that goes for time as well as treats.

■ *Respect your child's independence.* This is more challenging for parents of onlies. Why not just brush her teeth for her, since she's taking so long and you don't have another child who needs your help. Even at an early age, it's important to let her figure things out on her own, whether it's buttoning a shirt or figuring out how a toy works.

■ *If you respect your child's independence, she'll respect yours.* Onlies don't have to share Mom or Dad, and you may get used to giving your attention freely. But it's important to teach an only child that you have your own life, too.

For more information, see *Parenting an Only Child: The Joys and Challenges of Raising Your One and Only*, by Susan Newman, Ph.D. This book is filled with good advice for parents, lots of myth-busting facts about the singleton stereotype, and some fascinating studies on only children.

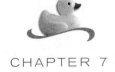

when accidents happen

what to do—and what not to do—when your child gets hurt

Y ears ago at a family gathering, a young relative fell to the ground and began having a full-body seizure. As doctors, my wife and I immediately went to his side—and promptly began debating over whether or not to put a wallet between his teeth. After all, aren't you supposed to put something between the teeth during a seizure? Actually, you should never do this (see the myth in this chapter on pages 229–231, for more). Our relative recovered with no intervention. Yet, the incident illustrated that when faced with emergency situations or first-aid questions, we may not be prepared with the latest information, or we may be too worried to think clearly—particularly if it's our own child who is hurting.

Obviously, if an accident is serious enough, your first move will be to call 911 and get help. But parents can be faced with medical emergencies that they must deal with on their own, at least until help arrives. What should they do first to help their child, or should they do anything at all? It's important to be armed with the facts—not the myths and misconceptions. On a less dire note, the average kid can get lots of boo-boos, and the average parent can get pretty good at making them feel "all better"—especially when their good intentions are backed by good (correct) information.

It's impossible to prevent all accidents, but it is possible to take preventive measures—and to be prepared, just in case.

Head Injuries
When (and why) to call a doctor

myth
If your child hits his head, keep him awake.

reality
With some monitoring, children can sleep safely.

the facts
Did you ever get conked on the head as a child, only to find that your mom's top priority was keeping you awake?

You didn't black out, it didn't really hurt, you weren't seeing double, there was not a drop of blood, but your mother was adamant that you stay as alert as a night-shift worker. Even to this day, many adults think that when a child (or anyone) gets any kind of bump on the head, allowing him to fall asleep is extremely dangerous to the brain. But if the head injury is not serious (I'll define those situations next), usually it's okay to let your child go to sleep, especially if he is still taking regular naps and is used to getting that midday rest, or if it's bedtime.

"Head trauma," "head injury," and "blow to the head" all sound very scary and painful—and they can be serious depending on the nature of the injuries sustained. But those are also phrases used to describe more minor thumps and bumps. Your child gets clocked on the head with a toy truck. He gets smacked by an errant rubber ball. He slips in his plastic swimming pool. Even when we take precautions, these kinds of things can happen. When does a bump on the head signal a more serious condition, such as a concussion or a head injury that requires a doctor's intervention without delay?

If any of the following conditions apply, contact your pediatrician immediately. Your child may be perfectly fine, but these symptoms might indicate a more serious head injury:

- You're dealing with a baby under age six months. Even a minor head bump can be serious for a young baby.

- Your child is unconscious for *any* amount of time, even seconds.

- Your child is confused; is having trouble talking (vocalizing for nontalkers), walking, or moving; shows signs of dizziness; is acting oddly (unusually irritable, very drowsy); or has convulsions (seizures) or unusual physical movements.

- There is bleeding or watery blood from the nose or ears. (Blood from the mouth may be from an injured lip, gum, or tooth.)

- You make any of these physical observations: Your child looks pale for more than an hour; his pupils appear to be different sizes; there is a visible indentation in the skull. This type of indentation could indicate a skull fracture. Note that even minor bumps on the head can cause "goose eggs"—but indentations are different.

- Your child complains of neck pain or severe headache. Children too young to describe their pain symptoms may cry excessively.

- Your child vomits more than twice.

If you visit the pediatrician, ask about allowing your child to sleep for uninterrupted stretches. If an injury was serious enough to warrant a trip to the doctor or emergency room, the doctor may recommend that you wake the sleeping child every two to three hours to make sure he is responsive (he wakes easily) and is behaving or verbalizing normally, and that he shows no signs of further injury. You should watch your child because signs of more serious head trauma, such as the symptoms in the bulleted list above, may not appear until hours or even days after the injury. You should also seek a doctor's guidelines on offering any pain medication.

If your child sustains a head injury and cannot get up on his own, do not move him (his neck or spine could be injured) and call 911.

Once again, use your parental common sense. Consider how he got hurt (what caused the injury; how great the impact was; if he fell a great distance onto a hard surface or fell onto soft ground; got hit by a heavy, hard object or by a soft one, and so on) and observe your child closely. If he is his normal, lively self, then he's probably okay. Most childhood bumps on the head are just that.

myth

If your child didn't black out after a fall, it's not serious.

reality

After a fall, your child can lose consciousness so briefly that you may not even notice.

the facts

It's possible to lose consciousness for seconds—such a short span of time that as an observer, you may not even notice. Any loss of consciousness due to a blow to the head indicates an interruption in normal brain function. Therefore, a child should always be checked by a doctor, even if the injury seemed minor and the loss of consciousnesses was momentary.

What if your child did not lose consciousness? It's still possible that she sustained a concussion, an injury to the brain that disrupts its normal functions. (A concussion is considered a "closed" head injury, meaning that nothing has penetrated the skull and there is no open wound. When there is no blood, we may be tempted to think there is no serious injury.) During a concussion, the brain literally gets jostled around in the skull, potentially causing bruising of the brain as well as nerve and blood vessel damage. Though that sounds horrendous, most concussions—which are more prevalent among older kids doing contact sports—are not serious. Though brain function is disrupted, the brain isn't necessarily damaged.

Concussions are often graded into three levels:

Grade 1 concussion Mild, no loss of consciousness. Your child is fine within twenty minutes of the injury or sooner.

Grade 2 concussion   No loss of consciousness, but more serious than Grade 1 because your child was slightly disoriented for more than twenty minutes after being injured. She may not recall what happened. See a doctor.

Grade 3 concussion   Loss of consciousness for a brief time. Your child may not recall what happened. See a doctor.

Most concussions are mild. However, if your child has any of the symptoms listed on pages 225–226 after a head injury, or if you're dealing with a child under six months of age—no matter how minor it may have seemed at the time—contact your doctor.

We may think of concussions as an injury that happens to school-age (often helmet-less) skateboarders, cyclists, soccer players, and other athletes; but babies, toddlers, and preschoolers can get them, too.

myth

It's okay for a child's bike helmet to have a little wiggle room.

reality

Helmets should fit snugly; this is one item you *don't* want your child to have to grow into.

the facts

Congratulations on making sure your new tricycle rider is wearing a protective safety helmet, but does it fit properly? It's not easy to fit a bike helmet on a squirming toddler, but it's important that the helmet fit snugly against the front and back of the head for the best protection. Don't use a hand-me-down from an older sibling or other child unless it fits correctly. (And don't use a helmet that has been in an accident; helmets should be replaced after accidents, even if there is no obvious damage.)

According to the Consumer Product Safety Commission (CPSC), a helmet can reduce the risk of head injury by 85 percent, and brain injury by 88 percent. Like car seats, helmets keep kids safer and can save lives, but if they don't fit properly, they don't do much good. Follow the manufacturer's instructions carefully when fitting your child's helmet, which should sit level on the head. It should not fall low on the forehead or tilt upward, nor should it move from side to side. The straps should fit comfortably but snugly under the chin. You don't want a helmet that will fall off or get knocked out of position during a collision.

The CPSC has a free, downloadable instruction booklet on choosing and fitting helmets, at http://www.cpsc .gov/cpscpub/pubs/349.pdf, and the Cincinnati Childrens' Hospital Medical Center also offers parents photos and step-by-step instructions on how to fit a helmet, at http://www.cincinnatichildrens.org/svc/alpha/r/bike-helmet/ fitting.htm.

Seizures
What (not) to do

myth
If your child has a seizure, place an object (such as a spoon or a wallet) into his mouth to prevent him from choking or swallowing his tongue.

reality
Do not put anything into his mouth.

the facts

For years, people believed that someone having a seizure could actually choke on or swallow his tongue, so a common practice was to insert something into the mouth—like a stick, a wallet, or a spoon. It is physically impossible, however, to swallow one's own tongue, even for a small child with a small tongue. In addition, observers of seizure are concerned that the person will bite his tongue; although this is not uncommon in a full-body seizure, if it happens at all it is when the seizure first begins. So by the time you see someone having a seizure, it is too late to prevent a tongue injury.

A relaxed tongue can block the airway in the mouth, however, so a child (or adult) having a seizure should be turned on his side, so that the tongue falls to the side of the mouth. The side-lying position also helps to drain oral secretions and prevent head injury. It's also advisable to place the hips higher than the head when the child is lying on her side, or to raise the child into a semi-sitting position, because while he can't swallow or choke on his tongue, he may choke if he vomits. Ironically, the old practice of inserting something into the mouth probably upped the risk of choking (on the object itself) or of damaging the teeth.

Seizures, also referred to as convulsions, are caused by abnormal electrical impulses in the brain. The resulting seizures or convulsions can take many forms, and they are often misunderstood. A generalized, tonic-clonic full-body seizure (or "grand mal convulsion") is just what it sounds like: arms and limbs twitch and flail with great force, and the child may lose consciousness. On the other end of the spectrum are tiny, almost unnoticeable convulsions, "petit mal seizures," also called "absence attacks," when a child appears to stare blankly and his attention cannot be gotten. (These can occur in children five and older; very young children do not get this type of seizure.) Eyelids may flutter, hands may move, he may exhibit other tics, or he may remain quite still.

He will have no memory of the incident; and it may take a while for adults to notice these seizures, as they can be as brief as a few seconds.

In addition, there are many variations on seizures between the grand mal and petit mal varieties; sometimes the muscles tense up dramatically, or they may relax entirely. "Epilepsy" describes a condition marked by recurrent seizures over a long period of time. Antiseizure medications can successfully control epilepsy.

Febrile convulsions (see pages 137–138) are the most common type of seizure among babies or young children. The likelihood of seizures declines with age, and children with absence attacks usually outgrow this condition, often without medication. If your child has any form of seizure, including a febrile convulsion, contact your pediatrician.

myth
You can make your child "snap out" of a seizure.

reality
You can keep the child safe, but you cannot halt the seizure.

the facts
The best thing you can do if your child has a seizure is to give her a safe environment. You can't get her to "snap out of it" by calling her name or touching her. A seizure is an electrical process in the brain, and you can't intervene with an internal process through external means.

A child who has a generalized seizure may be old enough to be embarrassed by the incident, especially since children will sometimes have a bowel or bladder accident immediately following this kind of seizure. They may also be frightened and disoriented, although they will have no memory of what they've just gone through. As an adult, you can be reassuring, compassionate, and protective of the child. Move furniture out of the way. Do not put anything in the child's mouth (see pages 229–231). Try to loosen any clothing, particularly around the neck, that may be constricting. You can be helpful in these ways, but you cannot stop the process from happening.

Cuts and Burns
First-aid care, and when to get more help

myth
Wounds need fresh air to heal.

reality
A covered wound heals more quickly and is less likely to leave a scar.

the facts
How many times do you remember scraping your knee on the playground and your mom suggesting you "air out" your battle wound? As you've already discovered for yourself, Mother didn't always know best, even if she made you a special milk shake after you sustained your cuts and scrapes. A covered wound will heal faster, with less scarring, than an uncovered one.

An ordinary bandage holds in the moisture, which prevents the skin from drying out and scabbing over. We tend to think of scabs as the body's natural and beneficial reaction to a wound, but in fact a scab actually slows down the healing process because it creates a barrier between the healthy cells and the damaged cells that need repair. Scabs also lead to an increased risk of scarring; and of course, if your child falls again on the unbandaged and unprotected area, he may reopen and increase the severity of the wound.

So if your little one gets a boo-boo, by all means kiss it—but first put a bandage on it.

myth
Treat a burn with an application of butter or ice.

reality
Don't treat burns with butter or ice.

the facts

If your child burns himself, stay away from the refrigerator and the freezer, but head for the faucet. The idea is to cool down the skin first (to relieve pain and swelling) by holding the burn under cool running water for about five minutes. Keep the water pressure low and gentle. You can also submerge a burned hand or finger in a pan of cool—not ice-cold—water, but the faucet may work best if the burn is on a forearm or other hard-to-submerge area. Putting ice on exposed, delicate skin tissue can actually cause frostbite. Butter or any oil-based substance, like petroleum jelly, traps heat. Do not put baking soda or any type of powder on the burn. See the following box for information on how to treat a minor burn at home.

When does a burn require a doctor's attention?

Burns vary in seriousness and should be treated accordingly. So how do you know if your child has a minor burn that you can treat at home, or something that requires a doctor's attention? Here's a quick guide, from mild to serious:

A *first-degree burn* is the least serious, causing redness and swelling but no blistering. (A mild sunburn, for instance, is a first-degree burn.) Still, a first-degree burn hurts and should be treated with cool water as soon as possible to relieve pain and swelling. You don't need to cover the burn or use any special creams, although some parents and pediatricians like pure aloe vera gels, which have cooling and moisturizing properties. First-degree burns don't leave scars when treated properly. If your child seems to be in pain from a first-degree burn even after topical treatments like those recommended above and is over six months old, you can offer over-the-counter pain relievers such as ibuprofen or acetaminophen.

A *second-degree burn* causes blistering; a doctor should be consulted for a burn that causes blisters, which can develop an infection. Loosely cover the blistered area with sterile gauze (a clean towel or sheet will do) until you can see a doctor. Note that blisters can take up to twenty-four hours to form, so a first-degree burn can become a second-degree burn. Second-degree burns cause a significant amount of pain and always require a doctor's attention and treatment. Do not pop any blisters, or infection may ensue. Second-degree burns could result in scarring.

A *third-degree burn* is where the skin is left white or charred, signaling serious tissue damage. In this instance, the skin is so badly burned away that blisters cannot form. This degree of burn is extremely serious and you should seek out a doctor, emergency room, or burn center immediately.

Seek medical attention if the burn is caused by electrical or chemical contact.

Bruises, Breaks, and Sprains
When sticks and stones hurt their bones

myth

If your child can wiggle or move an injured body part (such as a finger, an arm, a leg, or an ankle), the bone isn't broken.

reality

The "Can you move it?" test isn't the most effective way to rule out broken bones.

the facts

"Can you move it? Can you walk on it?"

It's actually possible to walk on a broken ankle or leg, and frequently on a broken toe. In fact, some bone breaks often go untreated because the injured person can put weight on or move the affected area.

If your child is injured but it does not seem serious (that is, it is not a reason to call 911 and a visual inspection does not show anything obvious, like a protrusion of bone or a deformed-looking bone), yet you aren't sure if it's a sprain or a break, get to a doctor as soon as possible for an X-ray.

The following signs may indicate a break:

- There was a snapping or grinding noise when the injury occurred.

- It's extremely painful (though it may be possible) for your child to move or put weight on the injured area.

- There is redness or swelling around the area, which may be bruised and tender to the touch; there is intense "point tenderness" when gentle pressure is applied to a specific part of the bone.

- The area looks abnormal (a limb is bent or can bend in an odd position).

Watch your child's reaction closely. I'm reminded of three children—all different ages—who recently suffered broken bones, each reacting in a distinct (age-appropriate, it would seem) way. A toddler fractured her wrist but did not cry excessively at the moment of injury, and eventually continued her playing; however, every time she put weight on her hand to get up from a sitting position she cried and whimpered. A first-grader collided with another child shin-to-shin playing soccer (without shin guards). He cried for about fifteen minutes and then stopped entirely, matter-of-factly insisting to all adults that his leg was broken. Because he could put weight on it, his parents did not think it was broken, nor did the ER doctor, but still the boy calmly insisted it was broken—and an X-ray proved that it was. A teenager fell off his skateboard and hurt his arm, mentioning it to his mom when she asked why he was holding his arm so stiffly. He did not think it hurt enough to merit a trip to the doctor, and she believed him. He walked around for a week with a fractured arm before he decided the pain wasn't getting any better and he no longer wanted to tough it out. (She regretted not pulling rank and dragging him to the ER right after it happened.)

The lesson each of these kids teach us is that broken bones aren't always obvious, and that it's best to get your child to a doctor as soon as possible if you're in doubt. The good news is that because children's bones are still growing, they are softer than those of a mature adult and they tend to "bend" more rather than break completely; and young children's bones can heal up to twice as fast as those of a teen or an adult.

myth

The best way to stop a bloody nose is to tilt the head back.

reality

Do not tilt the head back; keep it upright or slightly forward.

the facts

When a nosebleed starts suddenly, our instinct may be to tilt the child's head back, since our desire is to stop the blood from dripping out and downward. However, that position is a mistake because it can make blood flow into the throat, causing choking or vomiting. Instead:

- Have your child sit upright or lean slightly forward, and pinch the nostrils just below the bony bridge of the nose (you won't be able to detect much of a "bony bridge" in a young child, so just target the soft lower half of the nose).

- Apply firm pressure for a full ten minutes. Do not release pressure to see if the bleeding has stopped. (If your child is old enough, let her do this herself.)

- If the bleeding has not stopped, apply pressure for another ten minutes. If, after a second application of pressure, the bleeding continues, contact a doctor immediately.

Nosebleeds can be brought on by many things, including colds and allergies, or low humidity in the air. A child may insert something into the nose (including her own finger) and cause bleeding that way. A blow to the nose can also get the blood flowing. If your child gets frequent nosebleeds, particularly if you cannot pinpoint the cause, see your pediatrician.

Nosebleeds in children are not unusual and are usually harmless, but for the child (and the adult) they can be very unnerving because of the blood itself, as well as their sudden nature. Do your best to stay calm, since your child will take her cues from you.

The Great (Itchy) Outdoors
When bugs bite and plants are pests

myth
After a bee sting, don't squeeze out the stinger for fear of injecting additional venom.

reality

Remove the stinger as quickly as possible, by scraping or any other means.

the facts

Only honeybees leave a barbed stinger in place, and most "bee" stings are really from yellow jackets, which do not leave behind their stinger (and technically are wasps, not bees). If a bee's stinger is left in place, remove it as soon as possible, since additional venom can be pumped into the skin for thirty seconds or more after the bee has flown away. If possible, scrape the stinger (and the attached venom sac) with a long fingernail, a credit card, or the edge of a knife (carefully, if your child is squirming).

Although one is often cautioned that squeezing out the stinger will lead to additional venom being released into the skin, this may not be true. A recent study of timing and techniques for removing honeybee stings failed to find a difference in sting-induced swelling when scraping and squeezing methods were compared. The researchers also note that if the initial sting occurred because a honeybee was defending its nest, then it is important to leave the nest area immediately—since a chemical signal (an alarm pheromone) is also released with the sting, which tells other bees where the sting victim is and encourages them to also sting.

Most bee stings do not require medical attention, but see a doctor immediately if your child has difficulty breathing, seems weak or becomes unconscious, develops hives or has itching all over his body, is nauseated, or experiences swelling of the tongue, lips, or face.

myth

Insect repellent is safe for all children and babies.

reality

Do not use repellent on babies less than two months old, and choose repellents for children carefully.

the facts

Insect repellents have chemical components that make them effective, including DEET. Large amounts of DEET absorbed through the skin can be harmful, so choose products that contain no more than 10 percent to 30 percent DEET. A higher percentage means that the repellent is more effective; so if your child will be outside for a long time, choose a higher concentration of DEET. In addition to DEET, picaridin is also an effective component. It is odorless and considered less irritating than DEET. The AAP does not recommend the use of any insect repellents on babies younger than two months of age.

myth

Poison ivy can spread from person to person.

reality

There are many misconceptions about poison ivy, including that it's "contagious."

the facts

Your daughter is playing in the yard and kicks her ball into a hedge, running into the bushes to retrieve it over and over again. Later that night, she has a rash on her arms that she can't stop scratching, and a quick glance at the three-leafed vine growing at the base of the hedge confirms that the culprit is poison ivy. Should you keep her away from her siblings and other children? Should you go nuts washing everything (and everyone) she's touched? Should you worry when she gives you a good-night hug and wraps you in her arms?

First of all, an allergic reaction to poison ivy cannot be spread through the rash it causes or through the fluid in the blisters that come from the rash. Poison ivy (and its plant relatives, poison oak and poison sumac) contains an easily released resin or sap called urushiol, and brushing up against a sap-emitting plant is enough to cause a reaction in most people. Urushiol, which quickly binds to the skin, is released whenever the leaves or stems of the plant are torn or broken open; the plant is very fragile, so it doesn't take much to release the urushiol. Pets wander through poison ivy and get the substance on their fur, then bring it inside. (The animals themselves don't have a reaction.) And that ball your daughter was kicking? It has urushiol all over it. So do her socks and shoes.

You may wonder why, if she only got poison ivy on her arms, the next morning it appears to be spreading to other parts of her body. It may be because her arms had the greatest exposure to the urushiol when she picked up the ball, so the reaction was quicker and more apparent there. The severity of rash from poison ivy depends not only on how much oil was transferred to the skin but also which part of the body was exposed. Some parts of the body are more sensitive to the urushiol oil than others. Urushiol likes thinner skin it can penetrate, so while it may not affect the palms of the hands, the inner arms are a prime target.

Although the rash itself is not contagious, this is only true once the urushiol oil is washed off. Since urushiol oil remains active when transferred from one surface to another, it's possible to expose new areas of skin to urushiol if your child touched other parts of her body shortly after touching the area initially exposed to the oil. Shoes and socks, gardening tools, toys, clothing, or other objects (like pets, as mentioned) that come into contact with urushiol can also be the source of a later reaction. Amazingly, urushiol is so potent an irritant that five hundred people can develop a rash from the amount of oil on the head of a pin, and a half-tablespoon is all that is needed to give a rash to everyone on Earth!

According to the American Academy of Dermatology, about 85 percent of people exposed to poison ivy will have a reaction. However, most pediatricians don't see a lot of poison ivy in their young patients. This may be because patients are not likely to develop a rash following their initial exposure (though the rash will develop with subsequent exposures). The second reason is that babies and small children aren't usually playing on their own in areas where poison ivy grows. When kids are older, though, the risks increase as they follow their natural urges to explore new parts of the great outdoors—even that harmless-looking flower bed. Poison ivy, unfortunately, isn't limited to wilderness preserves.

If your child (or you) have been exposed to poison ivy, she's likely to have a reaction unless the skin is cleansed within about ten minutes. If you're lucky enough to catch it in that time frame, treat the skin immediately, preferably outside. Some dermatologists recommend cleansing first with rubbing alcohol and then rinsing with cool water. If you have no rubbing alcohol, rinse well with water—cold water from your garden hose will do. Then head inside and clean up with soap and warm water. If you use soap and water or a washcloth before rinsing the skin, the urushiol can stick to the soap or washcloth, and possibly spread further. Any clothing, toys, shoes, or other objects that have been in touch with urushiol should be thoroughly washed (use rubber gloves that you can toss afterward)—that goes for pets, too.

If you miss the ten-minute window and your child's reaction is severe, or if the rash affects the genital area, is near the mouth or eyes, or is widespread, see a doctor as soon as possible. Poison ivy can take days or, in some cases, one to two weeks to cause a reaction. The rash and blisters can last

two to three weeks, and it's usually an uncomfortable period.
Children may not be able to keep from scratching the blisters, which can get infected from germs on fingernails.
Time-tested treatments such as cold compresses, oatmeal
baths, and calamine lotion can bring some relief, and some
over-the-counter hydrocortisone creams may also work.

Urushiol does sound like something out of a bad horror
movie, with its ability to stick to Fido's or Snowball's fur and
its long "shelf-life" (urushiol can survive for years even in a
dead poison ivy plant, and people have been known to get
ill from inhaling smoke from burning the plants, so never
burn poison ivy). The best thing you can do is to learn to
identify poison ivy and keep your child away from it. (Try
the Internet for some up-close photographs; this is much
safer than doing your own field research. The following FDA
Web site is helpful: http://www.fda.gov/fdac/features/796_
ivy.html.) Though not impossible, it's very difficult to completely eradicate this stubborn plant from a yard or a garden,
as it must be completely removed and properly disposed of,
roots and all. (Unless your skin has superpowers, hire an
experienced landscaper to do the job.)

When your child is old enough to understand, show her
what poison ivy and its trouble-making cousins look like and
teach her to steer clear. The old warning "Leaves of three,
let them be" isn't a bad place to start.

Stopping Trouble in Its Tracks
Preventing accidents

myth

If your baby or child eats a poisonous substance, give her
syrup of ipecac right away to induce vomiting and get the
substance out of her system.

reality

Administering syrup of ipecac can actually do more harm than good in some cases, and should only be given if recommended by medical personnel.

the facts

It's true that many child care books will instruct you to have a first-aid kit at the ready for your toddler, and syrup of ipecac, which induces vomiting, was once considered one of the standbys in case your baby ingested a harmful substance. But giving your child the syrup may actually worsen the problem as well as her discomfort, particularly if she has ingested something that can burn or irritate the mouth, throat, or stomach. As emergency room workers say, "If the poison burns on the way down, it'll burn on the way up." And treating your child with syrup of ipecac may potentially conflict with other, more effective treatments, such as charcoal, in the ER. In some cases, the syrup can even have an undesirable sedative effect on a child.

If you suspect your baby has ingested something harmful, immediately call your local Poison Control center (1-800-222-1222), pediatrician, or emergency medical treatment center (it's a good idea to have these numbers posted near your phone). Follow their directions for treatment before you attempt to handle the situation on your own, as it all depends upon what your child has ingested. They may recommend you go to the nearest hospital or to your pediatrician for treatment, or they may in fact recommend the use of syrup of ipecac.

Prevention is the best course of action. Keep all harmful substances safely out of reach in baby-proofed cabinets, and keep a close eye on your little one once she starts crawling and mouthing objects. It's better to spend some time baby-proofing than to have to reach for that first-aid kit!

myth

You don't have to worry about drowning hazards at home if you don't have a backyard swimming pool.

reality

Children can drown in small amounts of water.

the facts

Sadly, every year children drown in bathtubs, buckets, toilets, and other open containers of water. While swimming pools are often fenced and gated, everyday water hazards within the home are often not seen as risks.

After car accidents, drowning is the leading cause of death among children between one and fourteen years old. While many drownings do happen in swimming pools (see the two water safety myths that follow), a child can get into a lot of trouble inside the home as well. A baby's or toddler's head is disproportionately heavy; if he leans over to explore an open container of water such as a bucket, or if he's curious about the toilet, it's easy for him to topple forward headfirst and get stuck. As part of your baby-proofing, keep toilet lids closed, and make sure there are no large open containers of water in your home such as buckets or full sinks. Even if you don't have a pool or are not near a large outdoor body of water, there are many other areas, such as decorative fountains or fishponds, rain barrels, ditches, and other water receptacles or collection areas that pose outdoor water hazards. Teach older siblings about drowning risks, inside and outside the home, that a young baby or toddler may face, since they may associate drowning only with swimming pools and other obvious outdoor recreational swimming areas, such as lakes, rivers, and beaches.

myth

"Water wings" or "floaties" will protect your child from drowning.

reality

Flotation devices can provide a false sense of security for both the child wearing them and the adult who should be in a supervising role; children can drown while using them.

the facts

Inflatable arm bands designed to help children float in the water are *not* lifesaving devices. Though they can help a child float, they will not stop her from going under the surface of the water and drowning. Never allow your child to use such flotation devices unless you are within an arm's length (defined as "touch supervision" by the AAP).

The AAP recommends that children not be given formal swim instruction until four years of age; although many children are exposed to swimming as babies and toddlers (and some can learn to swim), a child may not be developmentally ready for swimming lessons. Keep in mind that once your child does learn how to swim, she should still be supervised *at all times* when she is in or near the water; continue to practice touch supervision. Children who know how to swim can and do drown, even in shallow water.

myth

You will know when a child is drowning, or is in danger, because of the noise and commotion she will make.

reality

Drowning can happen quickly and silently.

the facts

Years ago, I stood at the edge of an in-ground swimming pool talking with a pediatrician friend of mine while her young daughter was on the verge of silently drowning, literally at our feet. It was incredibly frightening (fortunately, we noticed just in time and the child—now bound for college—was fine). The point is that we did not initially see—or hear—the event. If there are children in the water, be especially vigilant. Drowning can happen literally within seconds, and with no warning sounds such as audible shouts for help or loud splashing.

myth

Shopping carts with their built-in seats designed for children are safe.

reality

Even in a busy store, your child may be safer walking beside you or in a stroller than in a cart.

the facts

For decades children have ridden in shopping carts, and adults took this arrangement for granted, their biggest worry being that a child would sneak an extra box of cookies into the weekly grocery haul. However, each year thousands of kids are injured when shopping carts tip over, when they fall out of the cart, or if they become entrapped in the cart. Shopping carts typically tip when a child is trying to climb up or down the side of the basket, or while attempting to get into or out of the cart. Babies squirm and lean from side to side.

Toddlers try to stand up (even when they are belted into the cart's child seat) and climb out. Older children who don't fit in the child seat often try to ride, while holding on and standing outside the cart, or try to sit within the basket itself (involving climbing in and out of the cart, which is dangerous even if an adult helps). Older children push shopping carts holding younger siblings and cause accidents.

Shopping carts can be very unstable. Even if they are partially made of plastic, they can be extremely heavy, and if they are thrown off balance and topple over, the force and impact are significant. According to the AAP, more than twenty-four thousand children, most of them under five years of age, were treated at emergency rooms for various head and neck injuries associated with shopping carts in 2005.

Just because it seems designed to carry a child, that doesn't mean it's safe. In fact, the AAP now recommends children not be placed in carts and that parents look for other alternatives, such as having an older child walk, or using a stroller or wagon (or a Snugli-type front/back carrier for infants). Should you place your child in a cart, be aware of the risks and make sure you use the cart's seat belt or harness. Never allow your child to stand in the cart, ride in the basket, or ride outside the cart, and always assist or supervise your child getting into and out of the cart. Don't place infant carriers on the top of a cart (place them inside the basket), never leave a child alone in a cart, and don't let a child push a cart if another child is riding in it.

conclusion

I opened this book with a quote from John F. Kennedy, who reminds us that the biggest enemy of the truth is "very often not the lie . . . but the myth." Less than twenty years after he uttered those words, I was a brand-new medical student sitting in a large lecture hall, thrilled to be there, ready to learn, and prepared to absorb every bit of wisdom that was about to be imparted by these wise teachers in their crisp white coats. But instead of hearing profound and elegant thoughts on the art and science of practicing

medicine, here is how the dean of the medical school wel-
comed us: "Half of everything you are about to learn over
the course of your medical education is completely wrong,
but that's not the real problem. The problem is that we can't
tell you which half."

It didn't take long for me to realize the intent behind this
statement. Medical science is constantly evolving, and thus
many of the truths we are taught in medical school are relative,
not absolute. Back then we were certain that eating spicy foods
can lead to an ulcer and that babies are safest when sleeping
on their tummy. These weren't popular myths that medical
science dismissed; these were widely established truths, particularly in medical circles. It was only through solid medical
research and an open mind that physicians realized they were
wrong. As doctors, a large part of our job is to stay current with
the medical literature and the research, filter that knowledge,
and take away solid facts that we can apply to our decision
making, so that we can provide patients—including the youngest and the smallest among them, our children—with the best
solutions medical science can offer.

But, as you know from your own experience as a parent,
new medical information comes at us all the time, and it
often makes the headlines. We see "pediatrician-approved"
over-the-counter cough and cold remedies yanked from
drugstore shelves. We read that pregnant women do not
always need to avoid eating certain foods to reduce allergen
risks in their unborn children. We hear that the recommended age range for the flu vaccine gets extended to
the late teens—and college freshmen who live in dorms
are urged to get vaccinated for protection against bacterial
meningitis (suddenly, we may yearn for the colicky baby or
demanding toddler who seemed light years away from such
risks). The news is always breaking, but for every new fact
on children's health that emerges, a myth or a misunder-
standing is sure to follow.

Perhaps the public should be given the same message that I was given as a young medical student: half of the medical information that the media will share with you is wrong; we just don't yet know which half.

For instance, several years ago a well-known study documented a link between the incidence of nearsightedness and the use of night-lights (or overhead light while sleeping) for children under two. The findings were interesting enough to be reported by the media and found their way into newspapers and magazine across the country. As a result, untold numbers of parents took away the night-lights, thinking they were saving their children's eyesight. Then, a few years later, another study came along and disproved the link in a variety of ways, pointing out that the original study did not take into account whether or not the parents were nearsighted (this condition can be hereditary).

Even now, almost ten years after the original study was published and publicized by the media, it still causes confusion. (See pages 74–75, "Don't put your child to bed with a light on," for more information on this myth.) Unfortunately, sometimes the media reports one study—the exciting and newsworthy "new findings"—on a particular health topic but then ignores or underreports subsequent studies that may dispute or reinterpret the original findings. (A news editor may conclude that the topic has already been reported on.) Good scientists know that studies done just once cannot be considered conclusive. The studies must be replicated, but such third and fourth experiments are not nearly as interesting to the media as those first "new findings." Nor is the tenth study, which proves for the ninth consecutive time that only a tiny percentage of the general population is affected by the findings of that headline-grabbing first study.

The media isn't the only reason medical myths have a way of morphing into assumed facts. There is also our very human tendency to embrace the notion of "seeing is believing." We sometimes see what we want to see because that's what we've done our whole lives, and we ignore everything else (like science). We may be extremely fond of a dear grandparent who insisted we drink a cup of hot water with lemon juice to cure a headache. We swear we felt better after that hot drink, but did the lemon juice cure headache pain like Grandpa Dave claimed or was it the fact that we were encouraged to sit down, rest, and collect ourselves over a steaming mug of something that smelled nice? (Well, Grandpa Dave *did* have science in his corner, as the "placebo effect" is a well-documented phenomenon!)

Beyond the media and our own biases, it's not just that favorite relative, the well-meaning neighbor, or a child's preschool teacher who perpetuates a medical myth or offers a flawed interpretation of a fact, though these folks can regularly refresh the rumor mill (forgive any myth-maker who cares about your child, because their intentions are good). The old wives' tales have gone high-tech. The Internet is an excellent tool for keeping current on children's health—when it is used wisely. But it also creates conditions for a perfect storm of myth-making: when a new study or theory is presented, there is always someone ready with a real-time response. Never mind that the person or organization dispersing misinformation is unqualified or has an agenda. They have a Web site, a blog, an e-newsletter, and a send button. For parents, particularly those who are researching a pressing health concern on behalf of a child, it's a minefield of fact and fiction.

Even doctors and other health professionals aren't immune to subscribing to myths—either because of how information is reported in the literature (those "new findings" minus the follow-up studies), not keeping up with the literature (the reading only increases after medical school), or because the correct information has not been studied or publicized adequately. How many doctors still think spinach is a good source of iron? I would bet a lot still do, but the spinach myth was disproved years ago (see the myth "Spinach is a good source of iron" on pages 38–39.)

Where can you turn? Whom can you trust?

First of all, look at the source of the information. Who is telling you this, and why, and where—exactly—are they getting their information? Is there good science to back it up? How old is this information, and has it been updated in any way? Are there other reputable individuals or organizations that back this claim? Look at the AAP Web site (http://www.aap.org), for starters, or at other pediatric Web sites that you've come to like and trust. Look also at Web sites like the Centers for Disease Control and Prevention (http://www.cdc.gov/) or other not-for-profit Web sites where information is being disseminated in order to educate the public. (That's not to say that some for-profit Web sites don't do an excellent job, but if a Web site's reason for being is to sell you something, be wary.) Do some digging, use common sense as you examine the source, and—don't forget—talk to your pediatrician. Whether your concern is diaper rash or delayed speech, good pediatricians will help you sort through the information overload and highlight the "right" half. It's our job.

As you move out of the *BabyFacts* years and into later childhood, adolescence, and the teen years, you'll exchange myths on pacifiers for myths on topics ranging from chocolate and acne (Hershey bars don't cause zits) to the impact of video games (it depends on many things), skipping breakfast and weight-gain (so Mom was right—it really is the most important meal of the day), and knuckle-cracking among junior-high boys (no, it does not cause arthritis).

Right now, though, your child is years away from arguing with you about wearing a helmet while skateboarding. You'll be ready to win that one because you have the hard facts on head injury prevention and helmets (see pages 228–229—although you may have to buy him a cooler-looking helmet.) Yet, you may pick up the paper tomorrow and read a story on childhood asthma that raises more questions than it answers. Your child's best friend's grandmother may insist that macaroni and cheese soothes an upset tummy (and maybe it does for her grandchild because he's not nauseated—just hungry). You may stumble onto a Web site that claims tea-tree oil cures everything. Your head may spin and your eyes may cross as you try to separate fact from fiction in our information-based world.

But consider the source, ask the right questions, talk to your pediatrician, and remember that even if your eyes do cross, they won't get stuck. That one is most definitely a myth!

Index

absence attacks, 230–231
accidents, 223–224
  bruises/breaks/sprains,
    234–236
  cuts and burns, 232–234
  head injuries, 224–229
  insects and poison plants,
    237–242
  from mobile walkers,
    200–201
  prevention of, 242–247
  seizures, 229–232
  See also safety issues
acetaminophen, 125, 138–139
acetylsalicylic acid, 139
acne, 79
acute otitis media (AOM),
    142–144
Adesman, Andrew, 5–6
AIDS, 15
air cleaners, 161
alcohol
  consumed by nursing
    mothers, 10–12
  co-sleeping and, 70
Allerca cats, 157
allergies
  allergic conjunctivitis, 148

breast-feeding and, 16–17
to dust/dust mites, 160–161
eczema and, 97
heredity and, 154–156
organic foods and, 30
outgrowing, 159–160
to peanuts/nuts, 31–32
to pets, 156–158
seasonal, 158–159
"trigger foods" and, 30–31
See also asthma
American Academy of Pediatrics
    (AAP), 253
  on antibiotics, 143
  on autism, 152–153
  on body fat of children, 48
  on circumcision, 116, 117
  on dental care, 166
  on drowning prevention, 245
  on fluid intake, 18
  on fruit juice consumption,
    40–41
  on hearing evaluation,
    192–193
  on insect repellent, 239
  on iron, 21–22
  on milk consumption, 26, 28
  on mobile walkers, 200

American Academy of Pediatrics
(AAP) (*continued*)
on OTC medications,
123–124
on pacifier usage, 13
on poison ivy, 241
on spanking, 215
on sunscreen, 3–4, 93
on television watching,
197, 198
on thermometers, 135
on toilet training, 113
on vision evaluation, 195
on vitamin D, 35, 36–37
American Dental Association
(ADA), 166
"angel's kiss," 80–81
antibacterial soaps, 163–164
antibiotics, 126–127
for conjunctivitis, 148–149
for ear infection, 141–144
for strep throat, 146–147
antidepressants, 15
antidiarrheals, 108
antifungal ointment,
101–102
Appalachian State
University, 179
apple juice, 30
artificial sweeteners, 42–44, 45
aspartame, 42–44, 45
Asperger's Syndrome, 151,
152–154
aspirin, 15, 125, 139
asthma
eczema and, 30, 97
heredity and, 154–156
outgrowing, 159–160
See also allergies
attentiveness, of parents, 185

autism
Asperger's Syndrome, 151
myths about, 4
prevalence of autism spectrum disorders (ASDs),
152–154
axillary thermometers, 134–135

baby acne, 79
Babyfacts (Adesman), organization of book, 5–6
baby fat, 47–49
babyproofing, importance of,
243
"baby talk," 189–191
baby teeth, 164–165, 167. *See
also* teeth
baby wipes, 100–103
"Back to Sleep" educational
campaign, 53
bacteria, 121–122, 126–127
bacterial conjunctivitis,
148–149
ear infection and, 143
Barkley, Russell A., 213
bassinettes, 58–59, 69
bathing
cradle cap and, 85
earwax buildup and, 87–88
eczema and, 95–98
frequency of, 81–83
powder products and, 88–89
sponge bath for fever, 139
time of day for, 84–87
umbilical cord care and, 83
beds
bassinettes, 58–59, 69
bedtime routines and,
65–67
co-sleeping and, 67–71

transitioning from crib to bed, 71–74

bedtime routine, 65–66. *See also* sleep

bed-wetting, 118–120

bee stings, 237–238

behavior
discipline and, 210–212
gender as factor in, 217–219
of only children, 219–221
seeking help for problem behaviors, 212–213
sharing and, 213–215
spanking and, 215
working *vs.* stay-at-home mothers and, 216–217

belly. *See* stomach

Benton, Christine M., 213

bicycle helmets, 228–229

birth control, breast-feeding and, 18

birthmarks, 80–81

birth order
only children, 219–221
speech development and, 191–192

bisphenol A (BPA), 25

bladder problems, 174–175

blankets, for swaddling, 61

bleach, 129

bloody nose, 236–237

body fat, 47–49

body mass index (BMI), 48

bonding
breast-feeding *vs.* bottle-feeding, 19
co-sleeping and, 67–71

bones
broken, 234–236
vitamin D and, 36–37

books
brainpower and, 184
on discipline topics, 213
nearsightedness and, 198–199
on parenting only children, 221

bottle-feeding
baby teeth and, 167
at bedtime, 64–65
canned *vs.* concentrated formula, 19–21
cleaning equipment for, 22–23
iron in formula, 21–22
nipple confusion, 12–13
temperature of formula/milk, 23–25
See also breast-feeding

botulism, 42

bowel movements
color of, 109
constipation and, 107–109
diarrhea and, 171–172

boxes, as toys, 182

boys
behavior and gender issues, 217–219
circumcision of, 82–83, 116–117
peanut allergy in, 31–32
toilet training for, 115–117

BPA. *See* bisphenol A

brain
brain damage and fever, 136–137
brainpower and, 182–185
foreign language and, 185–186
head injuries and, 224–229

brain (*continued*)
    intelligence and, 178–180
    stimulation of, 180–182
breakouts. *See* rashes
breast-feeding
    allergies and, 16–17
    as birth control, 18
    bonding during, 19
    bowel movements and,
        107–108
    co-sleeping and, 68–69
    on demand, 8–9
    diaper rash and, 101
    diet of mother and, 10–14
    fluid intake and, 17–18
    foremilk and hindmilk, 9–10
    health of baby and, 15–16
    health of mother and, 14–15
    liquid intake and, 4
    nipple confusion, 12–13
    rubber band reminder
        method for, 10
    temperature of breast milk
        and nutrients, 25
    temperature of breast milk for
        bottle-feeding, 23–25
    vitamins in breast milk, 25,
        34–35
    See also bottle-feeding
breast infection (mastitis),
    14–15
breath-holding, for hiccups, 173
broad-spectrum sunscreen,
    93–94
bruises, 234–236
burns, 4–5, 233–234

cabbage, 11
"café au lait" marks, 81
caffeine, 12

calcium
    in cows' milk, 27
    needed by nursing
        mothers, 14
    vitamin D and, 36–37
calories
    from breast milk, 9–10
    junk food and, 33
    sugar in drinks, 46
canned (ready-to-feed) formula,
    19–21
carrots, 37–38
car seats, napping in, 61–62
Centers for Disease Control and
        Prevention (CDC), 253
    on breast-feeding and contra-
        indications, 15
    on immunization, 150, 152
changing diapers, 103–105,
    114. *See also* diapers
chicken soup, 130
child development, 177–178
    behavior and, 210–221
    brain and, 178–186
    physical growth and,
        206–209
    speech and hearing, 186–193
    vision and, 194–200
    walking, 200–206
childhood obesity
    artificial sweeteners and,
        43–44
    cows' milk and, 26–27
    sugar and, 46–49
chocolate, 12
cholesterol, 26, 47
Cincinnati Childrens' Hospital
        Medical Center, 229
circumcision, 82–83, 116–117
citrus juices, 39–40

Clark, Lynn, 213
classical music, 178–180
cloth diapers, 104, 105–107.
    See also diapers
clothing
    footwear and, 91–92,
        202–204, 205–206
    skin care and, 89–90
    sun exposure and, 92–95
    temperature and, 90–91
clotrimazole, 101–102
colds, 122–124, 127–130, 131,
    133, 152. See also illness
colic, 171–172
colostrum, 17–18
concentrated formula, 19–21
concussion, 227–228
conjunctivitis, 147–149
consciousness, loss of, 224–228
consonant sounds, 187
constipation, 107–109
Consumer Product Safety
    Commission (CPSC), 229
contraception, breast-feeding
    and, 18
convulsions. See seizures
cornstarch-based powder,
    88–89, 102
co-sleeping, 67–71
cosmetics, 29
cotton balls, 101
cotton swabs, 87–88
cough/cold remedies, 122–124
coughing, 129–130, 162–163
cows' milk
    consumption of, 27–28
    in diet of nursing mothers,
        13–14
    food allergies and, 17
    in formula, 20

hormones in, 28–30
introducing, 26–27
cradle cap, 85
crawling, 204–205
creams, for diaper rash,
    100–103
cribs
    mobiles for, 75
    positioning baby in, 52–54
    See also safety issues; sleep
crossed eyes, 194–195
"cruising," 205
cuts, 232–233

dairy
    mucus and, 133
    treating coughs/colds and,
        124–125, 133
    See also cows' milk
day care
    immunity and, 161–163
    toilet training and, 111
daytime wakefulness, 63–64
DEET, 239
dental care, 165–167
dentist visits, 166
DHA, 20
"diagnostic substitution," 153
"diaper-free" movement,
    112–113
diapers, 99–100
    bowel movements, color
        of, 109
    bowel movements and consti-
        pation, 107–109
    changing, 103–105, 114
    disposables vs. cloth, 104,
        105–107
    hygiene for wiping girls,
        174

diapers (*continued*)
  powder products, 88–89,
    102–103
  preventing/treating diaper
    rash and, 100–103, 169
  transitioning to dispos-
    able training pants, 112,
    113–114
  See also toilet training
diarrhea
  diet and, 171–172
  in nursing baby, 15–16
dietary fat
  in cows' milk, 26–27
  trans fats, 47
discipline
  punishment and picky
    eating, 34
  seeking help for problem
    behaviors, 212–213
  time-out technique, 210–212
disinfectant, 129
disposable diapers, 104,
  105–107. *See also* diapers
disposable training pants, 112,
  113–114
"double-jointedness," 209
dreams, fear of, 75–76
drowning hazards
  floatation devices and, 245
  lack of warning, 245–246
  in small amount of
    water, 244
drugs, co-sleeping and, 70
DTaP vaccine, 152
DTP (diphtheria, tetanus,
  pertussis) vaccine,
  151–152
dust/dust mites, allergies to,
  160–161

E. coli, 39
early-onset puberty, 28–30
ears
  cleaning earwax, 87–88
  ear infection, 141–147
  ear infection and teething,
    165
  taking temperature by,
    134–136
echinacea, 131
eczema, 95–97
  allergies and, 30
  bathing and, 97–98
emergencies. *See* accidents;
  illness; safety issues
environmental impact,
  of diapers, 106
epiglottis, 147
epilepsy, 231
erythema toxicum (ETN), 79
estrogen, 29
eustachian tubes, 142
Exersaucers (Evenflo), 201
eyes, 37–38
  eye contact, 184
  pinkeye (conjunctivitis),
    147–149
  vision development,
    194–200, 251

family bed, 67–71
farsightedness, 198–199
fat. *See* body fat; dietary fat
fears
  of dark, 74–75
  fever phobia and, 139–140
  of monsters, 75–76
febrile seizures, 137–138
feeding, 7–8
  allergies and, 16–17, 30–32

bottle-feeding, 12–13, 19–25,
    64–65, 167
breast-feeding, 4, 8–19,
    23–25, 34–35, 68–69, 101,
    107–108
cows' milk and, 26–30
diaper rash and introduction
    of solid foods, 101
diarrhea and, 171–172
diet and diarrhea, 171–172
diet and kidney stones, 174
fruit juices and, 18, 39–41,
    46
multivitamins and, 34–36
picky eating and, 32–34
sugars and, 41–49
vegetables, 37–38
vitamin D and, 36–37
See also individual names of
    foods
Ferber, Richard, 66–67
"Ferberizing," 66–67
fever
    febrile seizures and,
        137–138
    immunization and, 152
    outdoor play and, 140–141
    phobia of, 139–140
    reducers for, 138–139
    thermometers and, 134–136
    treating, 133–134
first-degree burns, 233–234
flexibility, 209
fluid intake
    chicken soup, 130
    diarrhea and, 171–172
    treating coughs/colds with,
        124–125
fluoride, 35–36, 166–167
focusing, 196

Food and Drug Administration
    (FDA)
    on poison plants (Web site),
        242
    on rBST, 29
    on trans fats, 47
food poisoning, 169–170
food sensitivity, 32
footwear, 91–92, 202–204,
    205–206
Forehand, Rex, 213
foreign language, 185–186
foremilk, 9–10
formula
    bowel movements and,
        107–108
    canned vs. concentrated,
        19–21
    vitamins in, 35
    warming, 23–25
    See also bottle-feeding
frozen milk/formula, 24–25
fruit juices, 39–41
    fluid intake by nursing baby
        and, 18
    sugar in, 46
fruits, 33

games, brainpower and, 184
garlic, 11
gauze pads, 166
gender, behavior and, 217–219
gentian violet, 83
giftedness, napping and, 57
girls
    behavior and gender issues,
        217–219
    early-onset puberty in, 28–30
    hygiene for wiping, 174
    toilet training for, 115–117

gland swelling, 144–145
glass, plastic vs., 24
grand mal convulsion, 230
"growing pains," 208
guardrails, 69–70, 72

hand-eye coordination, 75
hand sanitizer, 162–164
hand washing, 128–129
hay fever, 155–156
head injuries
    concussion from, 227–228
    helmets and, 228–229
    wakefulness and, 224–226
hearing evaluation, 192–193
hearing loss, 142, 192–193
heat rash, 79
height, 206–208
helmets, 228–229
hemangiomas, 81
HEPA air cleaners, 161
herbal cold/flu remedies, 131
heredity
    allergies and, 154–156
    height and, 206–208
    nearsightedness and, 251
    physical growth and,
        206–208
hiccups, 172–173
hindmilk, 9–10
HIV, 15
honey
    as cough remedy, 125
    as sweetener, 41–42
honey bee stings, 237–238
hormones
    baby acne and, 79
    in cows' milk, 28–30
    fever and, 137
housecleaning, 161

hydrogenated oils, 47
hyperactivity, 44–45
hypercarotenemia, 38
hypermobility, 209
"hypo-allergenic" cats, 157

ibuprofen, 125, 138–139
ice, burns and, 4–5, 233
illness
    allergies and asthma,
        154–164
    antibiotics for, 126–127
    baby teeth and, 164–168
    bacteria and, 121–122
    chicken soup for, 130
    colds, 127–130, 152
    conjunctivitis, 147–149
    dairy and mucus, 133
    ear infection and sore throats,
        141–147
    fever and, 133–141
    "growing pains," 208
    herbal cold/flu remedies, 131
    hiccups, 172–173
    immunization and, 4,
        149–154
    kidney stones, 173–175
    OTC children's cough/cold
        remedies for, 122–124
    reducing exposure to,
        161–164
    safe treatments for, 124–125
    stomach (tummy) problems,
        169–175
    viruses as cause of, 127–130
    vitamins and, 132
immunization, 4, 149–154
immunotherapy (allergy
    shots), 157
"infant potty training," 112–113

infants
    defined, for medication, 123
    defined, for purpose of book,
        6
    napping by, 58
    sleep patterns for, 56
    sunscreen for, 94
injuries. *See* accidents; illness;
        safety issues
insects
    repellent for, 238–239
    stings of, 237–238
intelligence, 178–180
interleukin, 137
intussusception, 169
iron, 21
    cows' milk and, 27–28
    in formula, 21–22
    in spinach, 38–39

joints, 209
Journal of Clinical
        Gastroenterology, 173

Kaiser Family Foundation, 197
kidney stones, 173–175

lactase, 17
lactose intolerance, 17
language
    brainpower and, 184
    delays in development of,
        186–188
    learning a foreign language,
        185–186
    See also speech development
laxatives, 108
"lazy eye," 194–195
LDL cholesterol, 47
lighting, 74–75, 199–200, 251

lisping, 188–189
listening, to children, 185
Long, Nicholas, 213
Lotrimin (clotrimazole),
        101–102
low-fat milk, 26–27
lymph glands, 144–145

"magic soap," 163–164
mango juice, 40
Manhattan Toy, 182
mastitis (breast infection),
        14–15
mattresses. *See* beds; cribs
medical science, evolving nature
        of, 250
medication
    acetaminophen and
        ibuprofen, 125, 138–139
    antibiotics, overuse of,
        126–127
    antibiotics for ear infection,
        141–144
    antibiotics for strep throat,
        146–147
    herbal cold/flu remedies and,
        131
    over-the-counter children's
        cough/cold remedies,
        122–124
    for respiratory allergies, 156
    used by nursing mothers,
        14–15
megadosing, of vitamins, 36
mercury (in vaccines), 4,
        151, 153
microwave, warming bottles
        in, 23–25
milaria rubra, 79
milia, 79

miliaria, 79
Miller, Zel, 180
mirrors, 181
MMR (measles, mumps, rubella) vaccine, 151
mobiles, for crib, 75
mobile walkers, 200–202
modeling by adults
  eating habits and, 33
  of pronunciation, 189–191
  toilet training and, 115–116
  See also parents
moisturizer, 98
monsters, fear of, 75
mothers
  diet of, and breast-feeding, 10–14
  health of, and breast-feeding, 14–15
  working *vs.* stay-at-home, 216–217
  See also breast-feeding; parents
"Mozart effect," 178–180
mucus, 126–127, 133
multivitamins
  for illness, 132
  need for, 34–36
music
  brainpower and, 184
  "Mozart effect," 178–180
Mycostatin, 101–102
myopia, 196–197

napping
  in car seats/strollers, 61–62
  daytime wakefulness and, 63–64
  need for, 57–58
  See also sleep
nasal allergies, 155–156

National Institutes of Child Health and Human Development, 216–217
National Institutes of Health, 37
nearsightedness, 198–199, 251
neurological development. *See* brain
newborns
  defined, 6
  napping by, 58 (*See also* sleep)
  positioning, for sleep, 5, 52–54, 60–61, 69
  sleep patterns of, 55–57
  See also feeding; skin care/ conditions; sleep
Newman, Susan, 221
"NICHD Study of Early Child Care and Youth Development (SECCYD) (National Institutes of Child Health and Human Development), 217
night, sleeping through, 62–63
night blindness, 38
nightlights, 74–75, 251
nightmares, 75–76
night terrors, 75–76
nighttime fears, 74–76
911, 224
nipples
  cleaning equipment for bottle-feeding, 22–23
  nipple confusion, 12–13
nosebleed, 236–237
nut allergies, 31–32
Nystatin, 101–102

obesity, co-sleeping and, 70
ointments, diaper rash, 100–103

on-demand feeding, 8–9
1-2-3 Magic (Phelan), 213
only children, 219–221
oral thermometers, 134–136
organic milk, 29–30
osteoporosis, 37
outdoor play
  brainpower and, 184
  illness and, 140–141
over-the-counter (OTC)
    remedies
  for cough/cold, 122–124
  for ear infection, 143
  for respiratory allergies, 156
  See also medication
ovulation, 18

pacifiers, 12–13
  sleeping position and, 53
  teeth and, 168
padded toilet seats, 111,
    117–118
Parenting an Only Child
    (Newman), 221
Parenting the Strong-Willed Child
    (Forehand, Long), 213
parents
  attentiveness of, 185
  bathing with babies, 86–87
  eating habits of, 33
  knowledge/myths about par-
    enting, 1–5, 249–254
  pronunciation by, 189–191
  sleep for parents of new-
    borns, 56
  toilet training and modeling
    by, 115–116
  working *vs.* stay-at-home
    mothers, 216–217
  See also breast-feeding;
    mothers

Pauling, Linus, 132
peanut allergy, 31–32
penile cancer, 116
petit mal convulsion, 230
pets
  allergies to, 156–158
  poison ivy and, 240, 241, 242
Phelan, Thomas W., 213
phthalates, 29
physical activity level, 48–49
physical growth
  "double-jointedness" and, 209
  "growing pains" and, 208
  heredity and, 206–208
picky eating, 32–34
pinkeye (conjunctivitis),
    147–149
plagycephaly, 54
plants
  poison ivy, 239–242
  seasonal allergies to, 158–159
plastic
  bisphenol A (BPA) in, 25
  glass *vs.*, for bottles, 24
  phthalates in, 29
plastic rings, as toys, 182
play
  outdoor play, 140–141, 184
  same-sex playmates and,
    218–219
  tummy time, 54
  See also child development
Poison Control (contact infor-
    mation), 243
poison ingestion, 242–243
poison ivy, 239–242
pollen, 158–159
pools, drowning danger of,
    244–246
port wine stains, 81
positional skull deformities, 54

positioning, for sleep, 5, 52–54,
    60–61, 69
potty chairs, 111, 117–118
powder, 88–89, 102–103
pregnancy, breast-feeding and,
    18–19
premature babies, 36
preschoolers
    defined, 6
    immunity and, 161–163
    napping by, 58
    sleep patterns for, 57
    sunscreen for, 94
    toilet training and, 111
prickly heat, 80
"progressive waiting"
    approach, 67
pronunciation, 189–191
protein, in cows' milk, 28
puberty, early-onset, 28–30
pull-on disposable training
    pants, 112, 113–114
pustular melanosis, 79

rashes
    diaper rash, 100–103, 165
    (See also diapers)
    eczema, 30, 95–97
    poison ivy, 239–242
    types of, 78–80
    See also skin care/conditions
rattles, 182
rBST, 29
reading
    brainpower and, 184
    nearsightedness and,
        198–199
ready-to-feed (canned) formula,
    19–21
rectal thermometers, 134–136

respiratory illness
    allergies and, 30, 154–161
    colds, 122–124, 127–130,
        131, 133, 152
    upper respiratory infection,
        126–127
    See also allergies; asthma;
        illness
restaurants, bottle warming
    in, 24
Reye's syndrome, 15, 125, 139
rhinovirus, 127–128
rice cereal, 64–65
rickets, 36–37
rings, for tub bathing, 86
Robb, John, 213
rubber band reminder method,
    for breast-feeding, 10
rubbing alcohol
    for poison ivy, 241
    umbilical cord care and, 83
"rule of quarters," 188

saccharin, 42–43
safety issues
    aspirin and Reye's syndrome,
        15, 125, 139
    during bathing, 85–87
    co-sleeping and, 68–70
    danger of syrup of ipecac,
        242–243
    drowning dangers, 244–246
    of helmets, 228–229
    of honey, 41–42, 125
    of mobile walkers, 200–202
    of packaging as toy, 182
    positioning for sleep, 5,
        52–54, 60–61, 69
    shopping carts and, 246–247
    See also accidents; illness

salicylates, 139
saline (saltwater) nose
    drops, 124
"salmon patches," 80–81
same-sex playmates, 218–219
scabs, 232–233
Schmitt, Barton, 139–140
Sears, William, 68
seasonal allergies, 158–159
seats, for tub bathing, 86
second-degree burns, 234
seizures, 137–138
    reacting to, 229–231
    stopping, 231–232
sentence development, 188
sharing, 213–215
shoes, 91–92, 202–204,
    205–206
shopping carts, 246–247
Sicherer, Scott, H., 31
side, sleeping on, 53–54, 60–61
singletons, 220
sippy cups, 188–189
sitting, 204
size of baby
    height and heredity, 206–208
    size/sleep correlation, 62–63
skim milk, 26–27
skin care/conditions, 77–78
    allergies and, 30
    bathing and, 81–83, 84–87
    birthmarks, 80–81
    clothing and, 89–92
    cradle cap, 85
    earwax buildup and, 87–88
    eczema, 30, 95–97
    poison ivy, 239–242
    powder and, 88–89, 102–103
    rashes and breakouts, 78–80
    sun exposure and, 92–95

umbilical cord care, 83
sleep, 51–52
    alcohol consumed by nursing
        mothers and, 12
    bassinettes for, 58–59, 69
    beds for, 71–74
    bedtime routines and,
        65–67
    bottles at bedtime and,
        64–65
    co-sleeping and, 67–71
    daytime wakefulness and,
        63–64
    diaper changing and,
        104–105
    "Ferberizing," 66–67
    illness and, 125
    napping and, 57–58, 61–62
    nighttime fears and, 74–76
    safe positioning for, 5, 52–54,
        60–61, 69
    sleep patterns and, 55–57,
        62–63
    swaddling and, 60–61
smoking, 70, 156
sneezing, 129–130, 162–163
soap, 82, 98
    antibacterial, 163–164
    hand sanitizer vs., 162–164
    laundry detergent, 79, 89
    for poison ivy, 241
    skin care and, 78
    types of, 163–164
socks, 91–92
soda, 40, 46
Solve Your Child's Sleep
    Problems (Ferber), 66–67
S.O.S. (Clark, Robb), 213
soy milk, 20
spanking, 215

speech development
  birth order and, 191–192
  hearing evaluation and,
    192–193
  language delays and,
    186–188
  lisping and sippy cups,
    188–189
  pronunciation and, 189–191
  speech therapy for, 191
SPF, in sunscreen, 93–94
spicy foods, 10–11
spinach, 38–39
sponge bathing, 82, 98, 139
sprains, 234–236
standing, 205
stay-at-home mothers, 216–217
steam, treating coughs/colds
    with, 124
stimulation, brain development
    and, 180–182
stings, 237–238
stomach
  colic, 171–172
  pain and kidney stones,
    173–175
  sleeping on, 5, 52–53, 69
  stomachache, 169–171
"stork bite," 80–81
strabismus, 194–195
"strawberry" hemangiomas, 81
strep throat, 145–147
strollers, napping in, 61–62
Sudden Infant Death Syndrome
    (SIDS), 13
  co-sleeping and, 68
  DTP vaccine and, 151–152
  safe positioning for sleep and,
    5, 52–54, 60–61, 69
  swaddling and, 60–61

sugar
  artificial sweeteners and,
    42–44, 45
  honey as substitute for,
    41–42
  hyperactivity and,
    44–45
  weight gain, 46–49
sunburn, 94–95
sunlight
  protection from, 92–95
  vitamin D and, 35, 92
sunscreen, 3–4, 37, 92–95
swimming pools, 244–246
swollen glands, 144–145
syrup of ipecac, danger of,
    242–243

talcum powder, 88–89, 102
taste buds, 32
teeth
  dental care, 165–167
  fluoride and, 35–36,
    166–167
  permanent, 167
  sugar and, 45
  teething, 164–165
  thumb-sucking/pacifiers
    and, 168
television
  exposure to, 197–198
  vision and, 196–197
temperature
  of bathwater, 84, 97
  "catching" cold and, 127
  layered clothing and,
    90–91
  nutrients in breast milk
    and, 25
  rashes and, 79–80

safety of, for bottle-feeding,
    23–25
for sponge bathing during
    fever, 139
swaddling and, 61
thimerosal, 4, 151, 153
third-degree burns, 234
throat infection, 145–147
thumb-sucking behavior, 168
time-out technique, 210–212
toddlers
    defined, 6
    dentist visits by, 166
    guardrails for, 72
    napping by, 58, 62
    sleep patterns for, 56–57
    sunscreen for, 94
toilet training
    bed-wetting and, 118–120
    of boys *vs.* girls, 115–117
    disposable training pants and,
        112, 113–114
    equipment for, 117–118
    hygiene for wiping girls, 174
    timing for, 109–113
    vocalizing and, 109
    See also diapers
toothbrushes, 166
toys
    brain stimulation and,
        180–182
    recommendations for,
        181–182
    sharing of, 213–215
trans fats, 47
"trigger foods," allergies and,
    30–31
tub bathing. *See* bathing
tympanic thermometers,
    134–136

umbilical cord care, 82–83, 83
University of California at
    Irvine, 179
unpasteurized juice, 40–41
upper respiratory infection,
    126–127
urinary tract
    infection (UTI), 116
    kidney stones and, 173–175
urushiol, 240–242
U.S. Consumer Product Safety
    Commission
    on co-sleeping, 68, 70
    on crib safety, 72

vaccines, 4, 149–154
vegetables, 37–38
    carrots, 37–38
    picky eating habits and, 33
    spinach, 38–39
vegetarians, nursing mothers
    as, 36
viruses
    illness and, 127–130
    viral conjunctivitis, 148–149
vision, 37–38
    crossed eyes and, 194–195
    lighting and, 199–200
    nearsightedness,
        198–199, 251
    television and, 196–197
vitamins
    in breast milk, 25
    for illness, 131, 132
    multivitamin supplements,
        34–36, 132
    vitamin A, 26, 38
    vitamin B_{12}, 27
    vitamin C, 36, 39–40,
        131, 132

vitamin D, 26, 27, 35,
36–37, 92
zinc, 36, 131
vocabulary
development of, 188
mispronunciation and,
189–191
vocalizing
during bowel movements,
108–109, 112
brainpower and, 184
speech development and, 187
vomiting, 172
by nursing baby, 15–16
poison ingestion and,
242–243
von Wolf, E., 39

wakefulness
head injuries and, 224–226
sleep patterns and, 63–64
walking
footwear and, 91–92,
202–204, 205–206
mobile walkers and, 200–202
stages of, 204–205
warm water method, for
bottles, 24
washcloths, 98, 101
wasps, 238

water
breast-feeding and, 4, 17–18
diluting fruit juices with, 41
fluid intake by nursing baby,
17–18
fluid intake by nursing
mother, 14
for poison ivy, 241
purification of, 22–23
treating coughs/colds with,
124–125
for treatment of burns,
4–5, 233
weight
childhood obesity, 26–27,
43–44, 46–49
of parent, co-sleeping and, 70
size/sleep correlation, 62–63
whole milk, 26–27
Whoozit (Manhattan Toy), 182
wipes, 100–103
working mothers, 216–217
wounds, treating, 232–234

yeast infection, 101–102
yellow jackets, 238
Your Defiant Child (Barkley,
Benton), 213

zinc, 36, 131